Listen to This!

By Linda G. Richman

Picture Symbols from *The Picture Communication Symbols Book I and II*
by Roxanna Johnson

Mayer-Johnson, Inc.
P.O. Box 1579
Solana Beach, CA 92075-7579
U.S.A.

Non-Speech Communication Products

First Printing September 1987
Second Printing January 1990
Third Printing August 1992
Fourth Printing November 1994
Fifth Printing May 1997
Sixth Printing May 1999
Seventh Printing October 2000

Printed in the U.S.A.

Mayer-Johnson, Inc.
P.O. Box 1579
Solana Beach, CA 92075-7579
U.S.A.

Phone: 800-588-4548 or 858-550-0084
Fax: 858-550-0449

ISBN 0-9609160-2-4

ABOUT THE AUTHOR

Linda G. Richman is a speech and language pathologist. She received her B.A. degree in Communication Sciences and Disorders from Montclair State College, and her M.S. degree in Speech Pathology from Syracuse University. She holds the certificate of Clinical Competence from the American Speech-Language-Hearing Association and has received the Governor's Teacher of the Year award in New Jersey. Ms. Richman works with multi-handicapped students, many of whom are nonverbal.

DEDICATION

To my family and friends
Who are supportive of me
And to my students
Who have made it all worthwhile

TABLE OF CONTENTS

Problem Solving

Auditory Memory

INTRODUCTION

Listen to This! is a book of comprehensive exercises for persons of all ages needing remediation in auditory processing skills. Originally designed for non-speaking people, these exercises have also proven successful with verbal clients having auditory processing deficits. It has been found that underlying auditory processing problems often limit the expressive abilities of both verbal and non-speaking persons. This makes it an important deficit to remediate. In addition, *Listen to This!* may serve as a general language activity program for lower functioning clients. It is recommended for use by special educators of all types, as well as anyone else working with clients demonstrating auditory processing disorders.

Auditory Processing Deficits: A Description

At first glance, verbal clients with auditory processing deficits may not appear to have a communication problem. They often are able to make socially appropriate comments and discuss events happening around them. It is not until they are asked specific questions, or are in a very structured language situation, that their communication problems become more evident. Often their word retrieval deficits and inability to sequence and generate subsequent thoughts become obvious. They may experience difficulty in comprehending, associating, and organizing what others are saying to them. Therefore, their responses become inadequate or inappropriate.

Non-speaking persons often experience the same type of auditory processing deficits. However, since the language output available to them is often so limited, it may not be as obvious. For instance, a "yes" or "no" answer is often all that is expected of them. They may be confused about what was said to them, but appear as if they understand when they answer "yes" or "no". Our usual focus with the non-speaking person is to increase their expressive abilities with augmentative means. However, when these clients have an additional auditory processing deficit, we should also focus on remediating this problem so that it won't limit expressive language growth.

Description of the *Listen to This!* Program

Listen to This! is divided into five chapters that correspond to some of the major problems contributing to auditory processing disorders. These are as follows:

Chapter 1, <u>Categorization</u>   This chapter is placed first because it forms a foundation for many auditory skills. Categorization exercises require knowledge of vocabulary and the ability to store vocabulary in logical groups. Once vocabulary is organized, it can be retrieved and used in associative and comparative thinking. Exercises in this chapter include:
- choosing one or more items that belong in a category
- determining a category name
- determining what does not belong in a category
- choosing items that fit in one category but not in a subcategory

Chapter 2, <u>Word Retrieval</u>   This chapter includes exercises requiring the client to comprehend what is said, think of the group of words associated with it, make comparisons, and then choose the one answer that is most appropriate. Exercises in this chapter include:
> - phrase and sentence completion with varying degrees of contextual cues
> - determining singular and plural referents
> - definitions of words (objects, people, and places)

Chapter 3, <u>Auditory Association</u>   This chapter provides opportunity for the client to comprehend the meaning of something said, associate the meaning of it with what they already know, and integrate it into a new meaning.   Exercises in this chapter include:
> - object associations
> - part/whole associations
> - analogies
> - questions

Chapter 4, <u>Problem Solving</u>   This chapter builds upon the earlier chapters. It uses categorization, word retrieval, association skills, and knowledge of cause and effect. Clients identify problems and determine solutions while:
> - completing if-then statements
> - making comparisons
> - determining missing or incorrect information
> - predicting outcomes
> - drawing conclusions

Chapter 5, <u>Auditory Memory</u>   This chapter gives clients practice in improving memory of auditory information through a series of progressively more difficult exercises. Expanding auditory memory capabilities aids clients in processing and retrieving longer pieces of information. Exercises in this chapter include:
> - recalling sequences of related items
> - recalling details from sentences and stories
> - following complex directions

Each page in the book is a separate exercise. Every page includes:
1. A title. This indicates the subcategory within the chapter.
2. Suggested directions. These are merely guidelines as each client will have different needs.
3. An objective. These may be helpful in writing IEP's for school-age children.
4. Picture symbols. These are used by the client to indicate his/her answers.
5. The actual questions, phrases, and sentences that comprise the exercise.

Suggestions for Using *Listen to This!*

All exercises in the book may be duplicated. This allows for each client to have his/her own page. Space is allowed on every exercise to write the client's answers. By duplicating a page twice (or sometimes more), you can also cut and paste the actual symbol answers on the pages. After finishing the exercise, the clients may then keep their worksheets for further practice. It may also be used as a reinforcement by allowing them to show others what they have accomplished that day.

The directions for each exercise are only guidelines. Each client will come with their own set of skills and limitations. Every exercise should be adapted to meet that individuals needs. To keep it a positive learning experience, a success ratio of at least 70% to 80% for each client is recommended. That means that some clients will need many prompts to evoke enough correct answers. Others will need few. Here are some examples of prompts which might be helpful: (1) giving the client the first sound of the word in question, (2) embellishing the information provided to give more clues to a particular word, (3) repeating the stimulus phrase or questions with emphasis on the important words, and (4) using a fill in the blank format.

The chapters have been arranged in a suggested order for presentation. Within each chapter there is some gradation from the simple to the more difficult. However, there is no definite order in which to present the exercises. Clients will have their own strength and weakness areas. These areas will guide you in determining which exercises are appropriate for an individual. Again, it is important to keep a high ratio of success for each individual.

Different clients will best indicate their answers to the exercises in different ways. Physically impaired persons may indicate their answer through various methods. They may be able to directly indicate their answers by pointing with a finger, a light beam, or head pointer. They may need to have someone scan the symbols for them and then indicate when the person has arrived at the correct symbol(s). All clients should be encouraged to say the word while they are indicating a symbol answer. Verbal clients may wish to simply say their answers rather than point.

Because of the simplicity of *Listen to This!,* parents and aides may successfully use the program. However, it is recommended that a trained professional monitor it s use. This is especially true in terms of choosing the appropriate exercises, types of prompts needed, how the client should indicate his/her answers, reinforcements to be used, etc.

The main emphasis of this program is to improve auditory processing. However, it is felt that the benefits may be more far reaching. Increased and more appropriate language output may be one result. Another potential benefit is that clients with symbol communication boards may feel more comfortable and motivated to use their boards. As they experience using picture symbols in exercises, rather than just on communication boards, they may begin to see that they are an acceptable, appropriate, and meaningful way to communicate.

Determining an Item in a Category

Directions: First review the symbols at the top of the page. Then have the client choose one picture from the top of the page to fit in each category as it is read.

Objective: The client will choose an item that belongs in a given category.

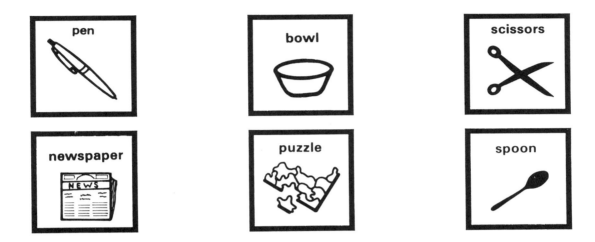

Choose:

a toy

something to cut with

silverware

something to write with

a dish

something to read

1

Determining an Item in a Category

Directions: First review the symbols at the top of the page. Then have the client choose one picture from the top of the page to fit in each category as it is read.

Objective: The client will choose an item that belongs in a given category.

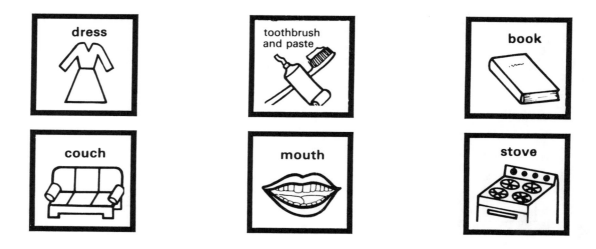

Choose:

something that belongs in the bathroom

something that belongs in the living room

clothes

something that belongs in the kitchen

something that belongs in school

part of the face

Determining an Item in a Category

Directions: First review the symbols at the top of the page. Then have the client choose one picture from the top of the page to fit in each category as it is read.

Objective: The client will choose an item that belongs in a given category.

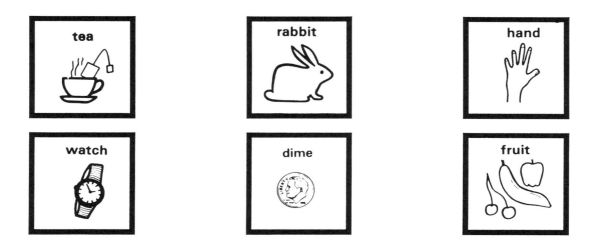

Choose:

something that you might pack in a picnic basket

a part of the body

an animal

a drink

something that tells time

money

3

Determining an Item in a Category

Directions: First review the symbols at the top of the page. Then have the client choose one picture from the top of the page to fit in each category as it is read.

Objective: The client will choose an item that belongs in a given category.

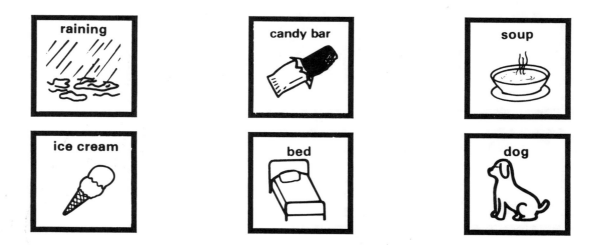

Choose:

a pet

something hot

something that belongs in a bedroom

a type of weather

something cold

candy

Determining an Item in a Category

Directions: First review the symbols at the top of the page. Then have the client choose one picture from the top of the page to fit in each category as it is read.

Objective: The client will choose an item that belongs in a given category.

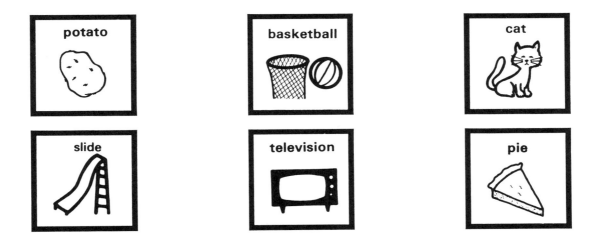

Choose:

something to turn on

a sport

something that belongs at a playground

a dessert

something soft

a vegetable

5

Determining an Item in a Category

Directions: First review the symbols at the top of the page. Then have the client choose one picture from the top of the page to fit in each category as it is read.

Objective: The client will choose an item that belongs in a given category.

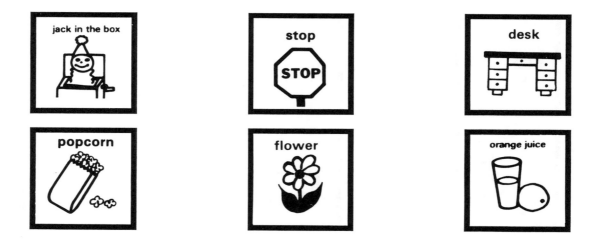

Choose:

something that grows

a snack

something that belongs in a classroom

a drink

something that belongs on a street

a toy

Determining an Item in a Category

Directions: First review the symbols at the top of the page. Then have the client choose one picture from the top of the page to fit in each category as it is read.

Objective: The client will choose an item that belongs in a given category.

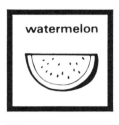
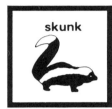
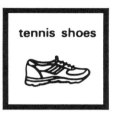

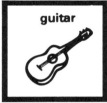
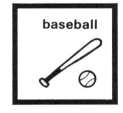
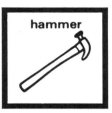

Choose:

something juicy

a tool

shoes

a sport

a musical instrument

an animal

7

Determining an Item in a Category

Directions: First review the symbols at the top of the page. Then have the client choose one picture from the top of the page to fit in each category as it is read.

Objective: The client will choose an item that belongs in a given category.

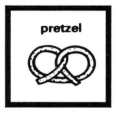

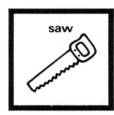

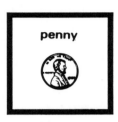

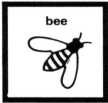

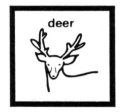

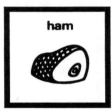

Choose:

money

an animal

a snack

a tool

an insect

meat

Determining Items in a Category

Directions: First review the symbols at the top of the page. Then have the client choose at least one picture from the top of the page to fit in each category as it is read. Each question has more than one answer. A picture can fit in more than one category.

Objective: The client will touch/name all of the items that belong in a given category.

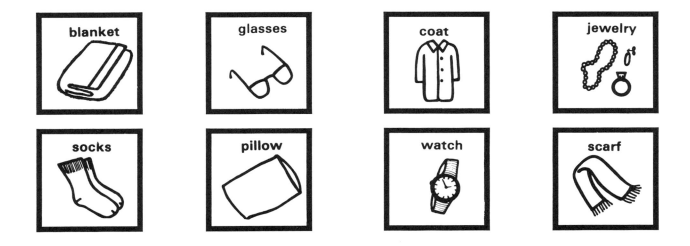

Choose:

everything we wear outside because it is cold

everything that is soft

everything that goes on a bed

all of the clothes

everything that is hard

everything we wear

Determining Items in a Category

Directions: First review the symbols at the top of the page. Then have the client choose at least one picture from the top of the page to fit in each category as it is read. Each question has more than one answer. A picture can fit in more than one category.

Objective: The client will touch/name all of the items that belong in a given category.

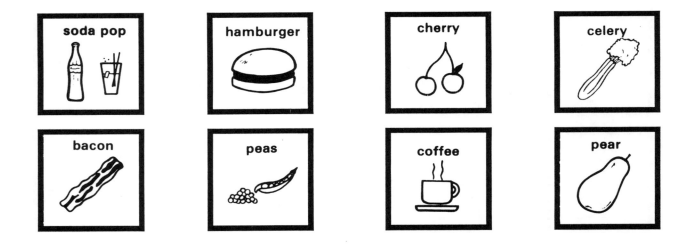

Choose:

all of the fruits

all of the meats

all of the vegetables

all of the drinks

all of the green foods

all of the cold foods and drinks

all of the warm/hot foods and drinks

Determining Items in a Category

Directions: First review the symbols at the top of the page. Then have the client choose at least one picture from the top of the page to fit in each category as it is read. Each question has more than one answer. A picture can fit in more than one category.

Objective: The client will touch/name all of the items that belong in a given category.

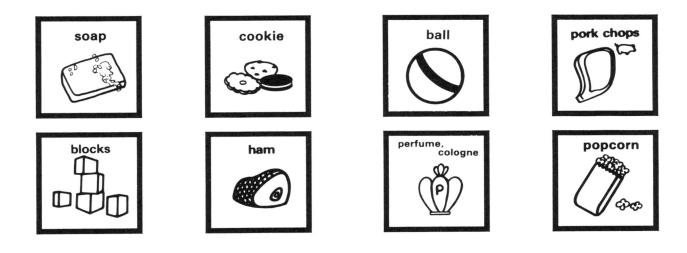

Choose:

all of the foods

everything that has a strong smell

all of the meats

all of the toys

all of the snacks

Determining Items in a Category

Directions: First review the symbols at the top of the page. Then have the client choose at least one picture from the top of the page to fit in each category as it is read. Each question has more than one answer. A picture can fit in more than one category.

Objective: The client will touch/name all of the items that belong in a given category.

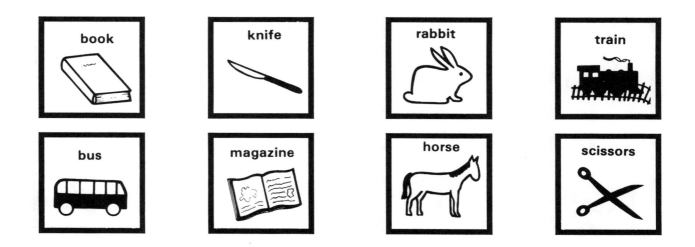

Choose:

everything that cuts

everything you can ride

everything that jumps

everything you can read

all of the animals

Determining Items in a Category

Directions: First review the symbols at the top of the page. Then have the client choose at least one picture from the top of the page to fit in each category as it is read. Each question has more than one answer. A picture can fit in more than one category.

Objective: The client will touch/name all of the items that belong in a given category.

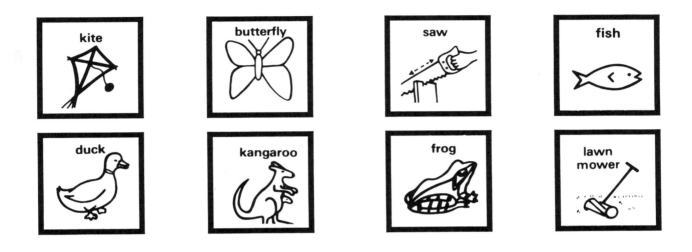

Choose:

everything that flies

everything that swims

everything that cuts

everything that is alive

everything that jumps

Name the Category

Directions: First review the symbols at the top of the page. The client listens to or reads each list of related items. Then the client chooses a picture from the top of the page to name the category which includes those items.

Objective: The client will determine the category after hearing a list of related items.

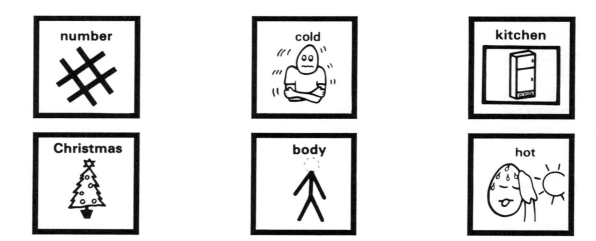

Choose:

ice cube - snow - refrigerator

tree - ornaments - Santa Claus

stove - fire - soup

nose - knee - shoulder

refrigerator - stove - dishes

8 - 4 - 3

Name the Category

Directions: First review the symbols at the top of the page. The client listens to or reads each list of related items. Then the client chooses a picture from the top of the page to name the category which includes those items.

Objective: The client will determine the category after hearing a list of related items.

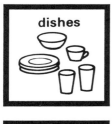
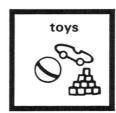
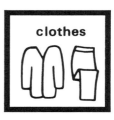

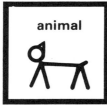
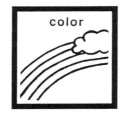
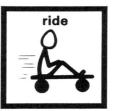

Choose:

orange - brown - black

tea set - electric train - doll

jacket - shirt - dress

bowl - cup - plate

kitty - puppy - lamb

boat - train - bicycle

Name the Category

Directions: First review the symbols at the top of the page. The client listens to or reads each list of related items. Then the client chooses a picture from the top of the page to name the category which includes those items.

Objective: The client will determine the category after hearing a list of related items.

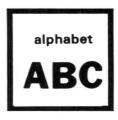
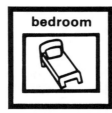
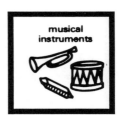

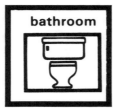

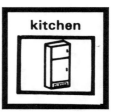

Choose:

dresser - bed - closet

shower - shampoo - towel

G - S - Q

sand - ocean - seashells

bells - drum - piano

pan - oven - food

Name the Category

Directions: First review the symbols at the top of the page. The client listens to or reads each list of related items. Then the client chooses a picture from the top of the page to name the category which includes those items.

Objective: The client will determine the category after hearing a list of related items.

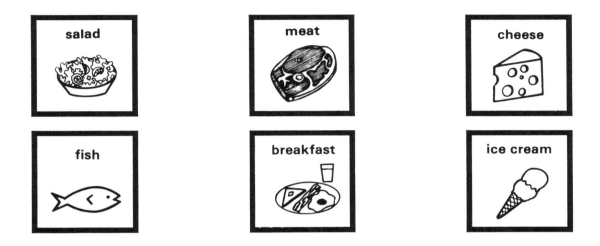

Choose:

ham - steak - bacon

lettuce - tomato - cucumber

cheddar - swiss - american

pancakes - eggs - cereal

halibut - goldfish - tuna

chocolate - vanilla - strawberry

Name the Category

Directions: First review the symbols at the top of the page. The client listens to or reads each list of related items. Then the client chooses a picture from the top of the page to name the category which includes those items.

Objective: The client will determine the category after hearing a list of related items.

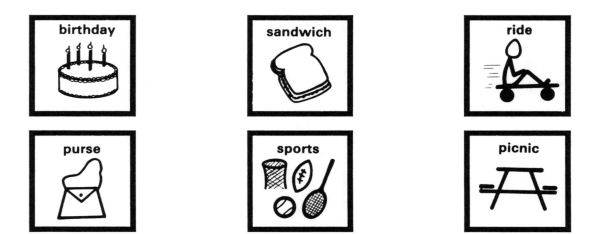

Choose:

baseball - tennis - basketball

basket - sandwiches - blanket

presents - cake - balloons

peanut butter and jelly - ham and cheese - egg salad

car - bus - plane

money - wallet - keys

Name the Category

Directions: First review the symbols at the top of the page. The client listens to or reads each list of related items. Then the client chooses a picture from the top of the page to name the category which includes those items.

Objective: The client will determine the category after hearing a list of related items.

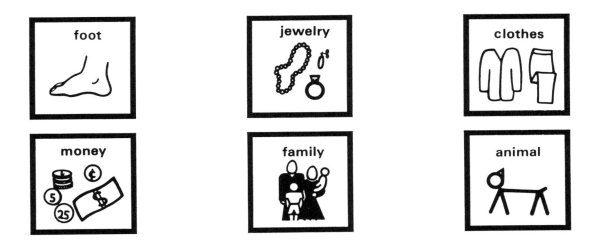

Choose:

socks - shoes - slippers

tiger - giraffe - kangaroo

pajamas - blouse - bathrobe

ring - necklace - bracelet

grandmother - aunt - father

dollar - penny - dime

Name the Category

Directions: First review the symbols at the top of the page. The client listens to or reads each list of related items. Then the client chooses a picture from the top of the page to name the category which includes those items.

Objective: The client will determine the category after hearing a list of related items.

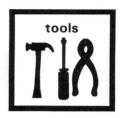 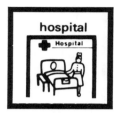 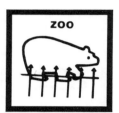

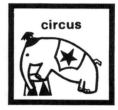 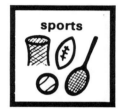 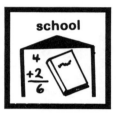

Choose:

hammer - screwdriver - saw

teacher - desk - blackboard

clown - tents - elephants

doctor - nurse - ambulance

football - baseball - hockey

monkeys - cages - giraffes

Name the Category

Directions: First review the symbols at the top of the page. The client listens to or reads each list of related items. Then the client chooses a picture from the top of the page to name the category which includes those items.

Objective: The client will determine the category after hearing a list of related items.

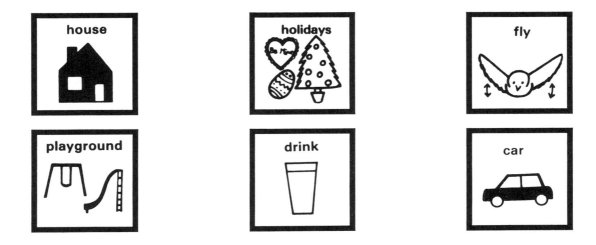

Choose:

windshield - wheels - doors

windows - walls - rooms

bird - bee - butterfly

Halloween - Thanksgiving - Lincoln's Birthday

swings - merry-go-round - jungle gym

coffee - hot chocolate - water

Name the Category

Directions: First review the symbols at the top of the page. The client listens to or reads each list of related items. Then the client chooses a picture from the top of the page to name the category which includes those items.

Objective: The client will determine the category after hearing a list of related items.

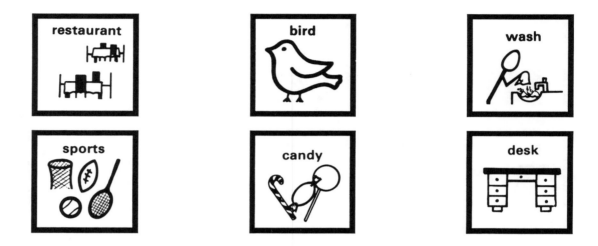

Choose:

menu - waitress - food

soap - detergent - shampoo

licorice - lollipop - jelly beans

football - golf - basketball

pens - paperclips - stapler

parakeet - robin - canary

Category Expansion

Directions: First review the symbols at the top and bottom of the page. The client chooses an appropriate category from below, after a list of related words is read. Then the client chooses one more item, from the top of the page, that will also fit in that category. More than one item may fit in the group, but the client needs to choose only one.

Objective: The client will determine the category, and name one more item that belongs in that category, after hearing a list of related items.

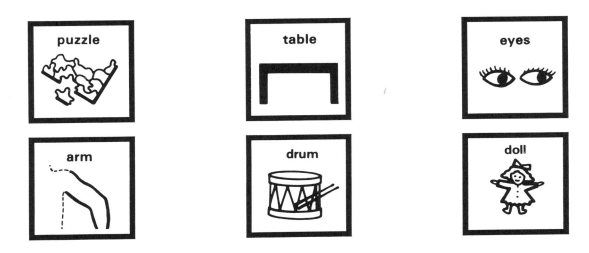

marbles - rocking horse - puppets

foot - back - stomach

bookcase - chest - chair

doll house - yo-yo - jump rope

horn - piano - guitar

leg - ear - hand

What is the category?

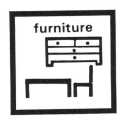
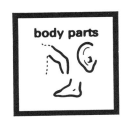
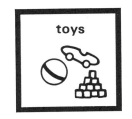
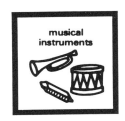

Category Expansion

Directions: First review the symbols at the top and bottom of the page. The client chooses an appropriate category from below, after a list of related words is read. Then the client chooses one more item, from the top of the page, that will also fit in that category. More than one item may fit in the group, but the client needs to choose only one.

Objective: The client will determine the category, and name one more item that belongs in that category, after hearing a list of related items.

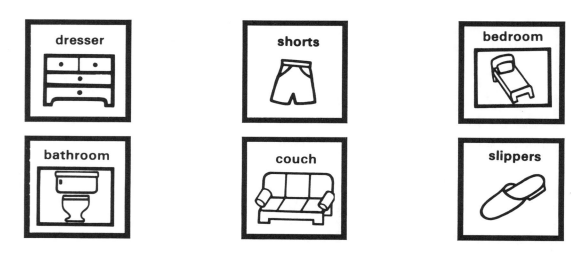

kitchen - living room - den

sandals - shoes - boots

chair - desk - lamp

dining room - playroom - basement

pants - bathing suit - coat

bed - table - cabinet

What is the category?

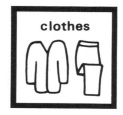 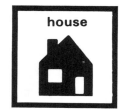 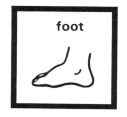 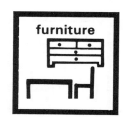

Category Expansion

Directions: First review the symbols at the top and bottom of the page. The client chooses an appropriate category from below, after a list of related words is read. Then the client chooses one more item, from the top of the page, that will also fit in that category. More than one item may fit in the group, but the client needs to choose only one.

Objective: The client will determine the category, and name one more item that belongs in that category, after hearing a list of related items.

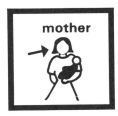
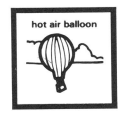
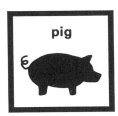
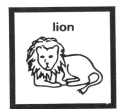
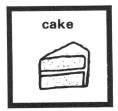
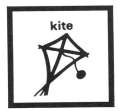

giraffe - bear - tiger

grandmother - uncle - brother

bird - jet - helicopter

chicken - lamb - cow

games - balloons - prizes

airplane - bee - rocket

What is the category?

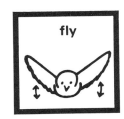
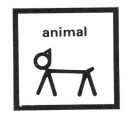

Category Expansion

Directions: First review the symbols at the top and bottom of the page. The client chooses an appropriate category from below, after a list of related words is read. Then the client chooses one more item, from the top of the page, that will also fit in that category. More than one item may fit in the group, but the client needs to choose only one.

Objective: The client will determine the category, and name one more item that belongs in that category, after hearing a list of related items.

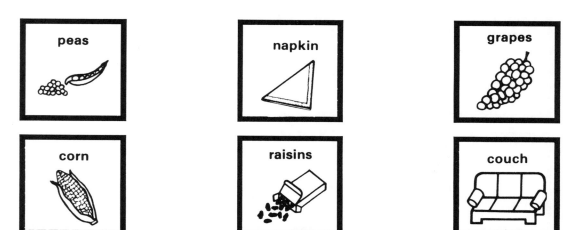

watermelon - peach - cherry

squash - cauliflower - carrots

green beans - broccoli - spinach

blanket - food - dishes

sofa - bench - chair

apple - banana - pear

What is the category?

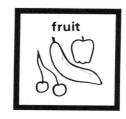 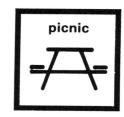 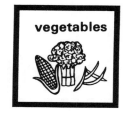 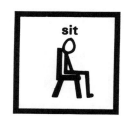

Category Expansion

Directions: First review the symbols at the top and bottom of the page. The client chooses an appropriate category from below, after a list of related words is read. Then the client chooses one more item, from the top of the page, that will also fit in that category. More than one item may fit in the group, but the client needs to choose only one.

Objective: The client will determine the category, and name one more item that belongs in that category, after hearing a list of related items.

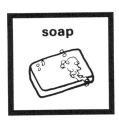
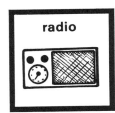

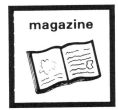
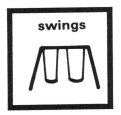
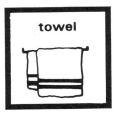

shower - mirror - razor

cartoons - baseball game - TV

merry-go-round - seesaw - slide

newspaper - book - letter

telephone - records - cassettes

bathtub - brush - comb

What is the category?

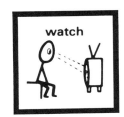
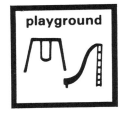
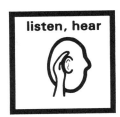

Category Expansion

Directions: First review the symbols at the top and bottom of the page. The client chooses an appropriate category from below, after a list of related words is read. Then the client chooses one more item, from the top of the page, that will also fit in that category. More than one item may fit in the group, but the client needs to choose only one.

Objective: The client will determine the category, and name one more item that belongs in that category, after hearing a list of related items.

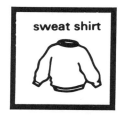
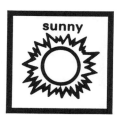
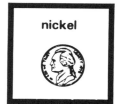
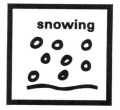
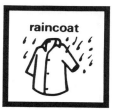

scarf - nightgown - suit

rainy - cloudy - foggy

pen - chalk - crayon

socks - jeans - skirt

dollar - penny - dime

sleet - windy - hot

What is the category?

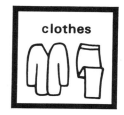
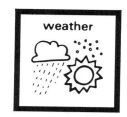
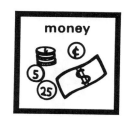

Determining What Does Not Belong

Directions: First review the symbols at the top of the page. To simplify the activity, point to the appropriate symbol at the bottom of the page. Then ask, "In the category of things to ride, which of the following words does not fit?" The client responds by choosing the picture at the top of the page. For more advanced clients, have them first choose the unrelated word and then the category of the related words at the bottom of the page.

Objective: The client will choose the item that does not belong within a list of related words.

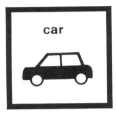
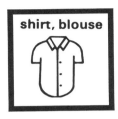

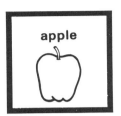

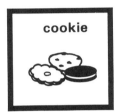
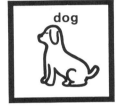
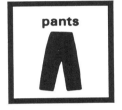
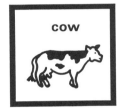

airplane - cow - bus - car

cookie - bread - apple - shirt

pants - dog - cow - cat

shirt - apple - socks - pants

bus - orange - soup - cheese

It doesn't belong because   it's not/you don't:

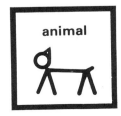
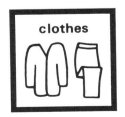
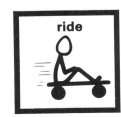

Determining What Does Not Belong

Directions: First review the symbols at the top of the page. To simplify the activity, point to the appropriate symbol at the bottom of the page. Then ask, "In the category of things to ride, which of the following words does not fit?" The client responds by choosing the picture at the top of the page. For more advanced clients, have them first choose the unrelated word and then the category of the related words at the bottom of the page.

Objective: The client will choose the item that does not belong within a list of related words.

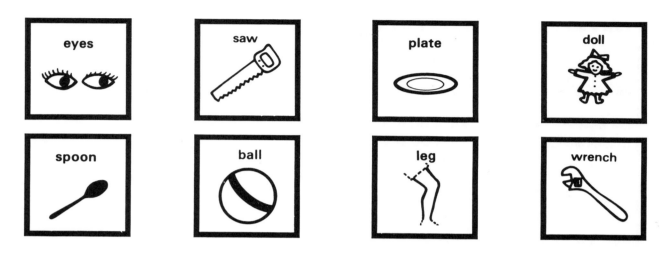

head - spoon - eyes - leg

cup - plate - saw - spoon

leg - ball - blocks - doll

saw - hammer - wrench - plate

eyes - ball - leg - nose

It doesn't belong because   it's not/you don't:

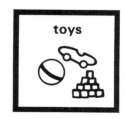 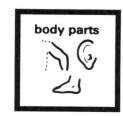 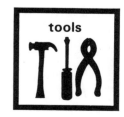 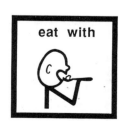

Determining What Does Not Belong

Directions: First review the symbols at the top of the page. To simplify the activity, point to the appropriate symbol at the bottom of the page. Then ask, "In the category of things to ride, which of the following words does not fit?" The client responds by choosing the picture at the top of the page. For more advanced clients, have them first choose the unrelated word and then the category of the related words at the bottom of the page.

Objective: The client will choose the item that does not belong within a list of related words.

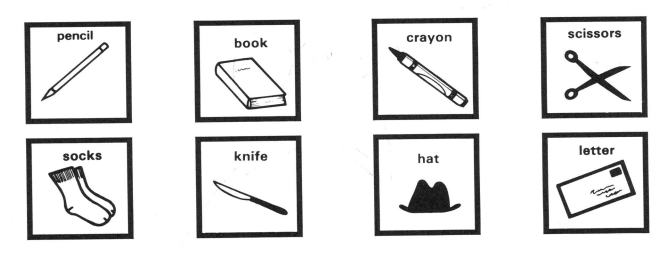

book - hat - coat - socks

letter - hat - newspaper - book

knife - saw - scissors - crayon

magic marker - crayon - letter - pencil

socks - boots - knife - hat

It doesn't belong because   it's not/you don't:

   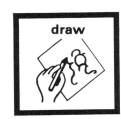

Determining What Does Not Belong

Directions: First review the symbols at the top of the page. To simplify the activity, point to the appropriate symbol at the bottom of the page. Then ask, "In the category of things to ride, which of the following words does not fit?" The client responds by choosing the picture at the top of the page. For more advanced clients, have them first choose the unrelated word and then the category of the related words at the bottom of the page.

Objective: The client will choose the item that does not belong within a list of related words.

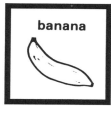 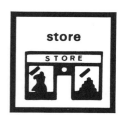 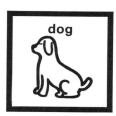 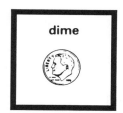

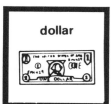 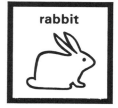 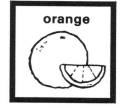 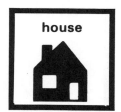

penny - dime - rabbit - dollar

apple - house - banana - orange

dog - sheep - rabbit - store

dollar - house - hotel - store

banana - dog - orange - grapes

It doesn't belong because   it's not/you don't:

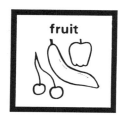 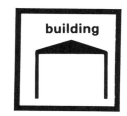 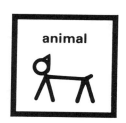 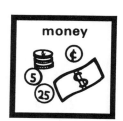

Determining What Does Not Belong

Directions: First review the symbols at the top of the page. To simplify the activity, point to the appropriate symbol at the bottom of the page. Then ask, "In the category of things to ride, which of the following words does not fit?" The client responds by choosing the picture at the top of the page. For more advanced clients, have them first choose the unrelated word and then the category of the related words at the bottom of the page.

Objective: The client will choose the item that does not belong within a list of related words.

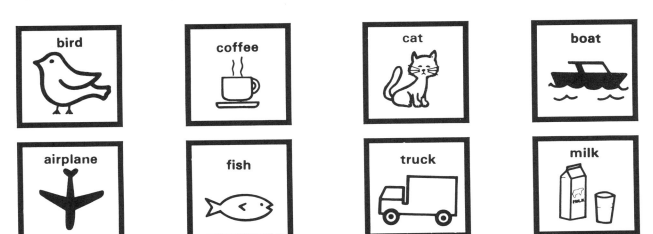

plane - butterfly - boat - bird

water - fish - coffee - milk

boat - truck - plane - bird

coffee - fish - submarine - boat

motorcycle - truck - cat - plane

It doesn't belong because   it's not/you don't:

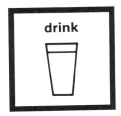
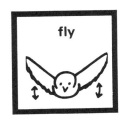

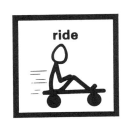

Determining What Does Not Belong

Directions: First review the symbols at the top of the page. To simplify the activity, point to the appropriate symbol at the bottom of the page. Then ask, "In the category of things to ride, which of the following words does not fit?" The client responds by choosing the picture at the top of the page. For more advanced clients, have them first choose the unrelated word and then the category of the related words at the bottom of the page.

Objective: The client will choose the item that does not belong within a list of related words.

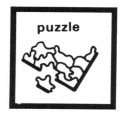
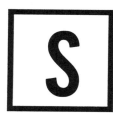
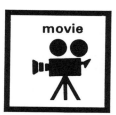
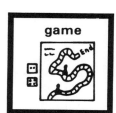
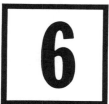
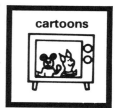
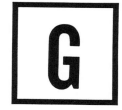
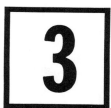

puzzle - movie - yo-yo - game

S - 3 - 2 - 6

TV - cartoons - movie - 3

A - G - 6 - S

game - blocks - cartoons - puzzle

It doesn't belong because   it's not/you don't:

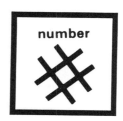
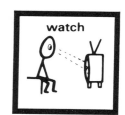
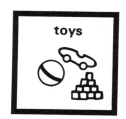
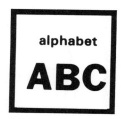

Determining What Does Not Belong

Directions: First review the symbols at the top of the page. To simplify the activity, point to the appropriate symbol at the bottom of the page. Then ask, "In the category of things to ride, which of the following words does not fit?" The client responds by choosing the picture at the top of the page. For more advanced clients, have them first choose the unrelated word and then the category of the related words at the bottom of the page.

Objective: The client will choose the item that does not belong within a list of related words.

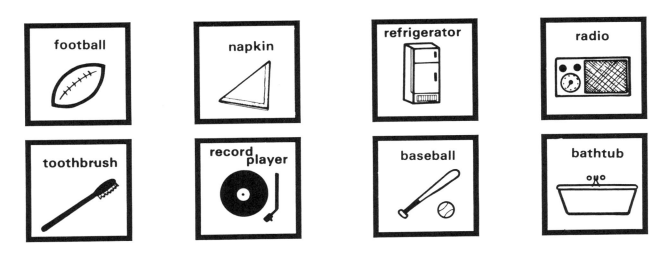

toothbrush - mirror - refrigerator - bathtub

music - record player - radio - baseball

toothbrush - knife - refrigerator - napkin

baseball - record player - football - golf

comb - napkin - toothbrush - bathtub

It doesn't belong because   it's not/you don't:

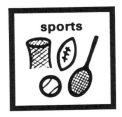 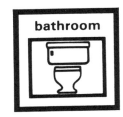 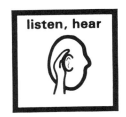 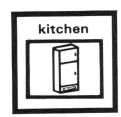

35

Category Exclusion

Directions: First review the symbols at the top of the page. The client chooses the pictures from the top of the page that fit in the given category but do not include the last item stated.

Objective: The client will choose the items that belong with a given category, but not within the subcategory stated.

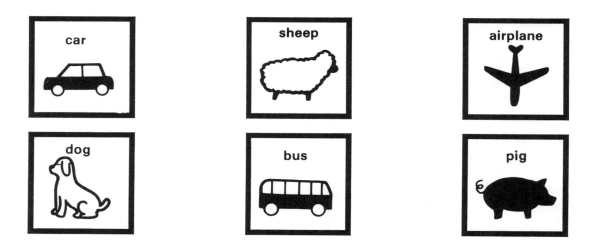

Touch all the animals except dog.

Touch all the vehicles except car.

Touch all the animals except pig.

Touch all the vehicles except bus.

Touch all the animals except sheep.

Touch all the vehicles except airplane.

Category Exclusion

Directions: First review the symbols at the top of the page. The client chooses the pictures from the top of the page that fit in the given category but do not include the last item stated.

Objective: The client will choose the items that belong with a given category, but not within the subcategory stated.

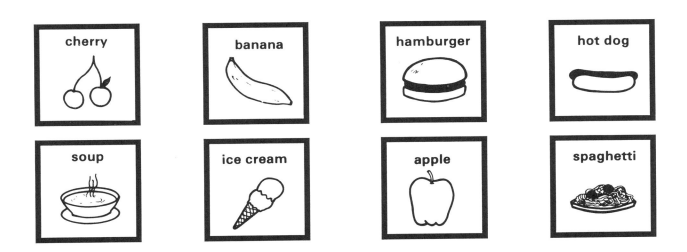

Touch all the fruits except apple.

Touch all the foods except fruit.

Touch all the cold foods except banana.

Touch all the hot foods except spaghetti.

Touch all the foods except meat.

Touch all the foods except the cold ones.

Category Exclusion

Directions: First review the symbols at the top of the page. The client chooses the pictures from the top of the page that fit in the given category but do not include the last item stated.

Objective: The client will choose the items that belong with a given category, but not within the subcategory stated.

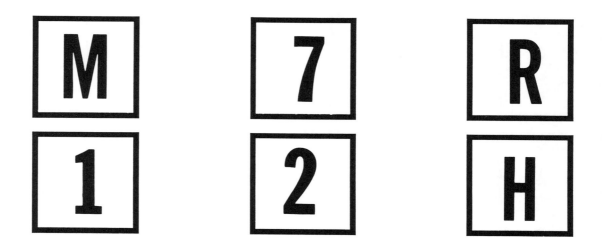

Touch all the letters except M.

Touch all the numbers except 7.

Touch all the letters except H.

Touch all the numbers except 1.

Touch all the letters except R.

Touch all the numbers except 2.

Category Exclusion

Directions: First review the symbols at the top of the page. The client chooses the picture from the top of the page that fits in the category stated, but does not fit in the subcategory.

Objective: The client will choose the item that belongs in the given category or exhibits the given attribute, but is exclusive of the subcategory given.

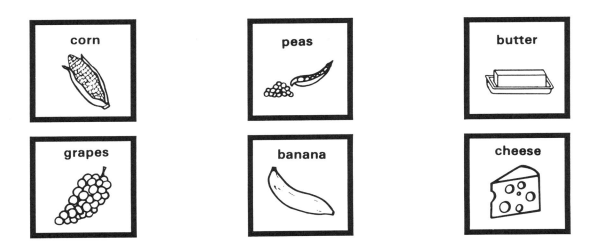

It's a vegetable, but it's not peas.

It's a fruit, but it's not grapes.

It's a fruit, but it's not yellow.

It's yellow, but it's not a fruit or vegetable.

It's a vegetable, but it's not yellow.

It's a dairy product, but it's not butter.

Category Exclusion

Directions: First review the symbols at the top of the page. The client chooses the picture from the top of the page that fits in the category stated, but does not fit in the subcategory.

Objective: The client will choose the item that belongs in the given category or exhibits the given attribute, but is exclusive of the subcategory given.

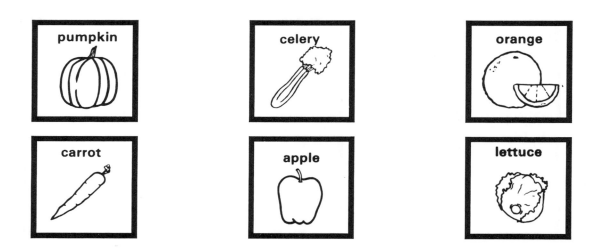

It's a fruit, but it's not orange.

It's a vegetable, but it's not green.

It's round, but it's not orange.

It's a vegetable, but it's not a carrot or lettuce.

It's orange, but it's not a carrot or an orange.

It's a fruit and it's orange, but it's not a pumpkin.

40

Category Exclusion

Directions: First review the symbols at the top of the page. The client chooses the picture from the top of the page that fits in the category stated, but does not fit in the subcategory.

Objective: The client will choose the item that belongs in the given category or exhibits the given attribute, but is exclusive of the subcategory given.

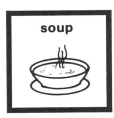

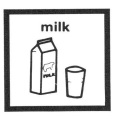

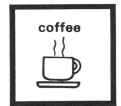

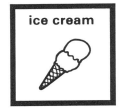

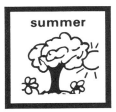

It's a drink, but it's not hot.

It's a food, but it's not cold.

It's hot, but it's not a food or drink.

It's a season, but it's not hot.

It's a drink, but it's not cold.

It's cold, but it's not milk or winter.

Category Exclusion

Directions: First review the symbols at the top of the page. The client chooses the picture from the top of the page that fits in the category stated, but does not fit in the subcategory.

Objective: The client will choose the item that belongs in the given category or exhibits the given attribute, but is exclusive of the subcategory given.

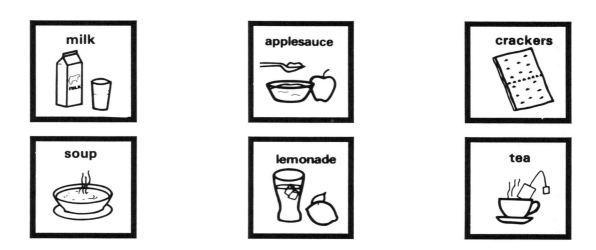

It's hot, but it's not a drink.

It's a drink, but it's not cold.

It's a drink and it's cold, but it's not milk.

It's a food, but it's not hot or crunchy.

It's a food, but it's not hot or mushy.

It's a drink, but it's not lemonade or tea.

42

Category Exclusion

Directions: First review the symbols at the top of the page. The client chooses the picture from the top of the page that fits in the category stated, but does not fit in the subcategory.

Objective: The client will choose the item that belongs in the given category or exhibits the given attribute, but is exclusive of the subcategory given.

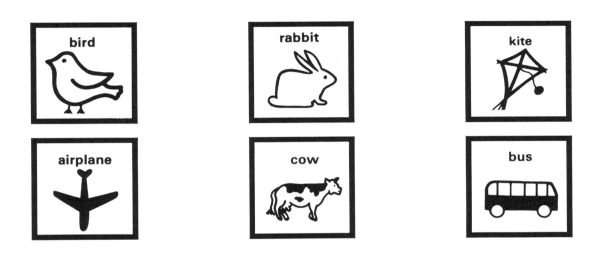

It flies, but it doesn't have wings.

It's heavy and it flies, but it's not an animal.

It's an animal that doesn't fly and it's not heavy.

It flies, but it's not a toy or a vehicle.

It's an animal, but it doesn't fly.

It's a vehicle, but it doesn't fly.

43

Category Exclusion

Directions: First review the symbols at the top of the page. The client chooses the picture from the top of the page that fits in the category stated, but does not fit in the subcategory.

Objective: The client will choose the item that belongs in the given category or exhibits the given attribute, but is exclusive of the subcategory given.

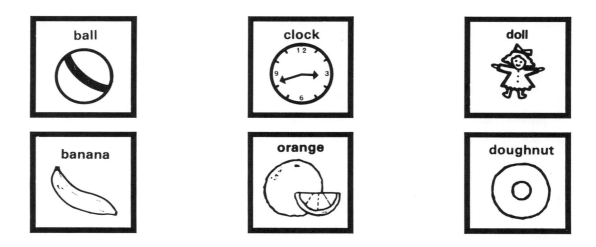

It's a toy, but it's not round.

It's a fruit, but it's not round.

It's round, but it's not a food or a toy.

It's a food and it's round, but it's not a fruit.

It's a fruit, but it's not a banana.

It's round, but it's not a clock or food.

Category Exclusion

Directions: First review the symbols at the top of the page. The client chooses the picture from the top of the page that fits in the category stated, but does not fit in the subcategory.

Objective: The client will choose the item that belongs in the given category or exhibits the given attribute, but is exclusive of the subcategory given.

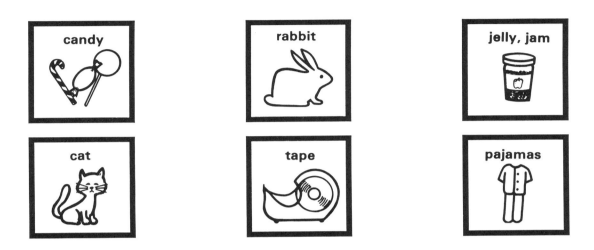

It's sticky, but it's not food.

It's an animal and it's soft, but it's not a cat.

It's soft, but it's not an animal.

It's a food and it's sticky, but it's not candy.

It's soft, but it's not clothes or a rabbit.

It's sticky, but it's not tape or jelly.

Final Verb Phrase Completion

Directions: First review the symbols at the top of the page. The client chooses a symbol to fill in the blank as each phrase is read. Some phrases may have more than one correct answer.

Objective: The client will choose the appropriate item(s) to complete a verb phrase.

radio	light	bell	door
ball	television	window	present

Shut the _____.

Catch the _____.

Turn on the _____.

Ring the _____.

Open the _____.

Throw the _____.

Final Verb Phrase Completion

Directions: First review the symbols at the top of the page. The client chooses a symbol to fill in the blank as each phrase is read. Some phrases may have more than one correct answer.

Objective: The client will choose the appropriate item(s) to complete a verb phrase.

dishes	fish	flower	face
plant	hair	hand	dog

Feed the _____.

Water the _____.

Comb your _____.

Dry the _____.

Wash your _____.

Clap your _____.

Final Verb Phrase Completion

Directions: First review the symbols at the top of the page. The client chooses a symbol to fill in the blank as each phrase is read. Some phrases may have more than one correct answer.

Objective: The client will choose the appropriate item(s) to complete a verb phrase.

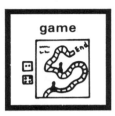

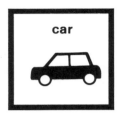

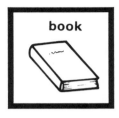

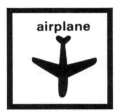

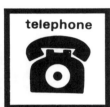

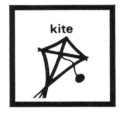

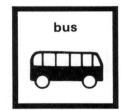

Sharpen the _____.

Drive a _____.

Read a _____.

Play a _____.

Fly a/an _____.

Answer the _____.

Final Verb Phrase Completion

Directions: First review the symbols at the top of the page. The client chooses a symbol to fill in the blank as each phrase is read. Some phrases may have more than one correct answer.

Objective: The client will choose the appropriate item(s) to complete a verb phrase.

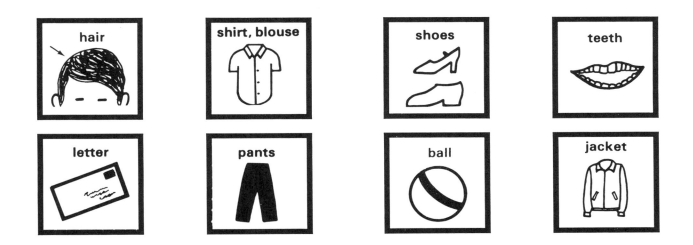

Zip your _____.

Kick the _____.

Brush your _____.

Write a _____.

Button your _____.

Tie your _____.

49

Noun Phrase Completion

Directions: First review the symbols at the top of the page. The client chooses a symbol to fill in the blank as each phrase is read. One or two symbols will be left over and not used as answers.

Objective: The client will choose the appropriate item(s) to complete a noun phrase.

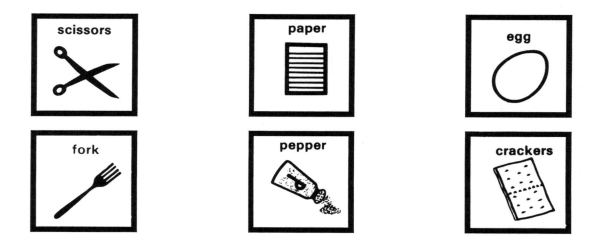

cheese and _____

bacon and _____

pencil and _____

knife and _____

salt and _____

Noun Phrase Completion

Directions: First review the symbols at the top of the page. The client chooses a symbol to fill in the blank as each phrase is read. One or two symbols will be left over and not used as answers.

Objective: The client will choose the appropriate item(s) to complete a noun phrase.

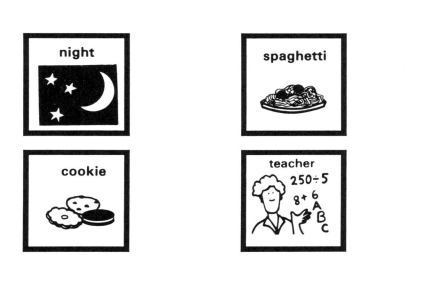

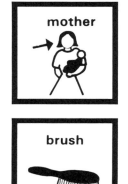

milk and _____

meatballs and _____

comb and _____

day and _____

father and _____

Noun Phrase Completion

Directions: First review the symbols at the top of the page. The client chooses a symbol to fill in the blank as each phrase is read. One or two symbols will be left over and not used as answers.

Objective: The client will choose the appropriate item(s) to complete a noun phrase.

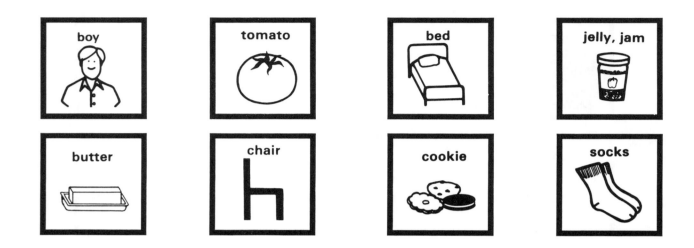

bread and _____

table and _____

girl and _____

peanut butter and _____

shoes and _____

lettuce and _____

Noun Phrase Completion

Directions: First review the symbols at the top of the page. The client chooses a symbol to fill in the blank as each phrase is read. Some phrases may have more than one correct answer.

Objective: The client will choose the appropriate item(s) to complete a noun phrase.

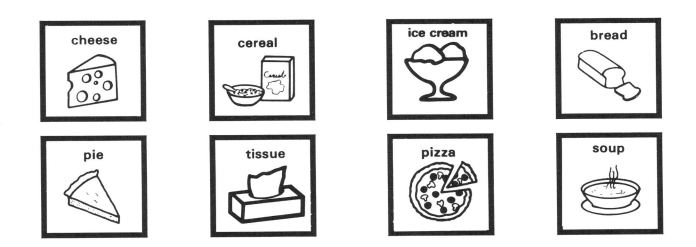

A bowl of _____.

A loaf of _____.

A box of _____.

A slice of _____.

A scoop of _____.

Noun Phrase Completion

Directions: First review the symbols at the top of the page. The client chooses a symbol to fill in the blank as each phrase is read. Some phrases may have more than one correct answer.

Objective: The client will choose the appropriate item(s) to complete a noun phrase.

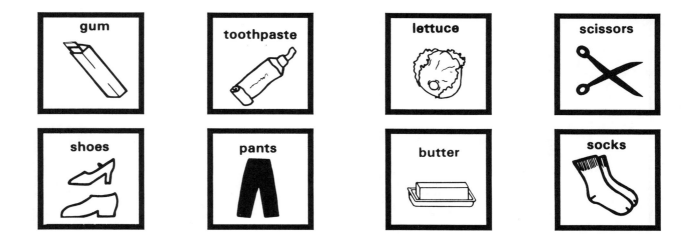

A pair of _____.

A stick of _____.

A tube of _____.

A pack of _____.

A head of _____.

Noun Phrase Completion

Directions: First review the symbols at the top of the page. The client chooses a symbol to fill in the blank as each phrase is read. Some phrases may have more than one correct answer.

Objective: The client will choose the appropriate item(s) to complete a noun phrase.

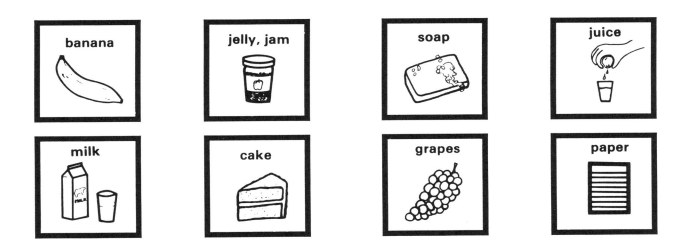

A piece of _____.

A glass of _____.

A jar of _____.

A bunch of _____.

A sheet of _____.

A bar of _____.

Initial Verb Phrase Completion

Directions: First review the symbols at the top of the page. The client chooses a symbol to fill in the blank as each phrase is read. Some phrases may have more than one correct answer. Use the first one as an example.

Objective: The client will choose the appropriate action to complete a verb phrase.

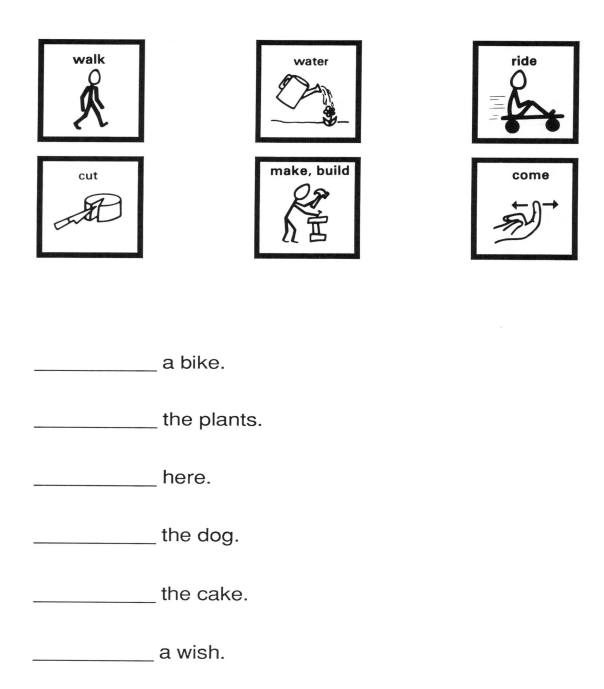

_____ a bike.

_____ the plants.

_____ here.

_____ the dog.

_____ the cake.

_____ a wish.

Initial Verb Phrase Completion

Directions: First review the symbols at the top of the page. The client chooses a symbol to fill in the blank as each phrase is read. Some phrases may have more than one correct answer. Use the first one as an example.

Objective: The client will choose the appropriate action to complete a verb phrase.

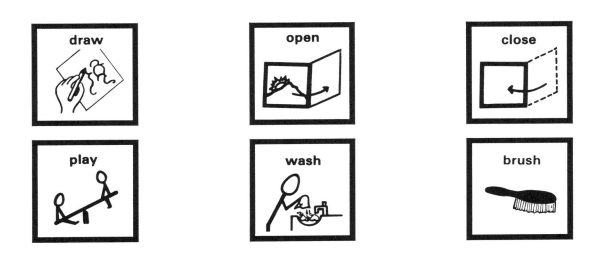

_____ your eyes.

_____ your hair.

_____ a picture.

_____ a game.

_____ the door.

_____ your hands.

Initial Verb Phrase Completion

Directions: First review the symbols at the top of the page. The client chooses a symbol to fill in the blank as each phrase is read. Some phrases may have more than one correct answer. Use the first one as an example.

Objective: The client will choose the appropriate action to complete a verb phrase.

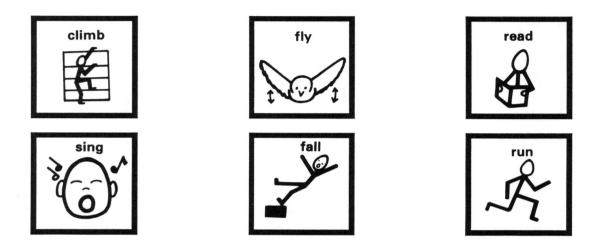

_____ a song.

_____ a race.

_____ a story.

_____ a kite.

_____ a ladder.

_____ down.

Initial Verb Phrase Completion

Directions: First review the symbols at the top of the page. The client chooses a symbol to fill in the blank as each phrase is read. Some phrases may have more than one correct answer. Use the first one as an example.

Objective: The client will choose the appropriate action to complete a verb phrase.

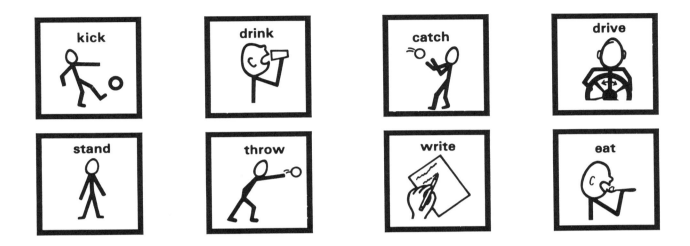

_____ the car.

_____ the ball.

_____ up.

_____ your lunch.

_____ a letter.

_____ your milk.

Initial Verb Phrase Completion

Directions: First review the symbols at the top of the page. The client chooses a symbol to fill in the blank as each phrase is read. Some phrases may have more than one correct answer. Use the first one as an example.

Objective: The client will choose the appropriate action to complete a verb phrase.

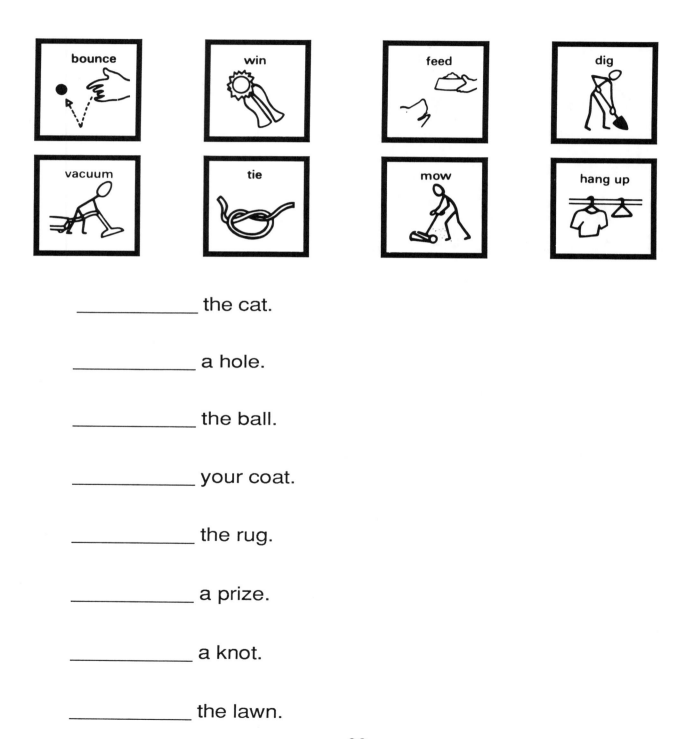

_____ the cat.

_____ a hole.

_____ the ball.

_____ your coat.

_____ the rug.

_____ a prize.

_____ a knot.

_____ the lawn.

Naming an Object

Directions: First review the symbols at the top of the page. The client chooses a symbol as each description is read.

Objective: After hearing a statement of an object's function and/or characteristics, the client will name the object.

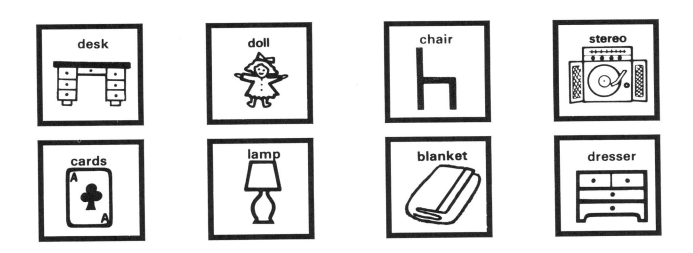

It's on your bed. It's a cover.

You play games with these.

You keep clothes in it.

You turn it on. It gives you light.

You sit on it.

You need this to play records.

Children play with it.

You do work at this.

Naming an Object

Directions: First review the symbols at the top of the page. The client chooses a symbol as each description is read.

Objective: After hearing a statement of an object's function and/or characteristics, the client will name the object.

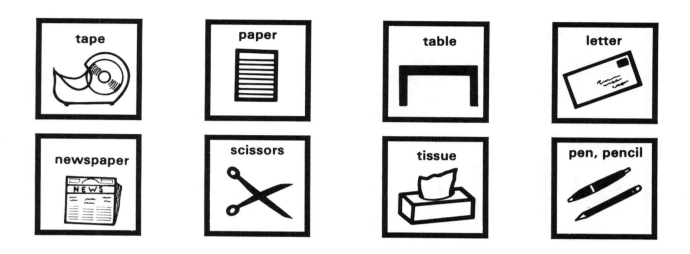

It's sticky. It holds paper together.

It' something you get in the mail.

You need this to cut paper.

You sit at this. It's a piece of furniture.

It's something you read.

You blow your nose in it.

You write on this.

You write with these.

Naming an Object

Directions: First review the symbols at the top of the page. The client chooses a symbol as each description is read.

Objective: After hearing a statement of an object's function and/or characteristics, the client will name the object.

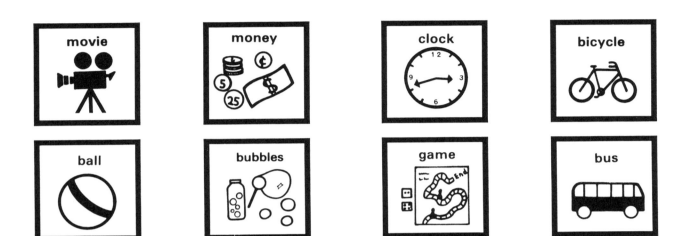

It's round. You throw it. You bounce it. You catch it.

Many people ride in this at the same time.

It's something you watch in the theater.

You ride it. It has two wheels.

You need it to buy things.

It shows you the time.

You can blow these in the air.

It's something you play.

63

Naming an Object

Directions: First review the symbols at the top of the page. The client chooses a symbol as each description is read.

Objective: After hearing a statement of an object's function and/or characteristics, the client will name the object.

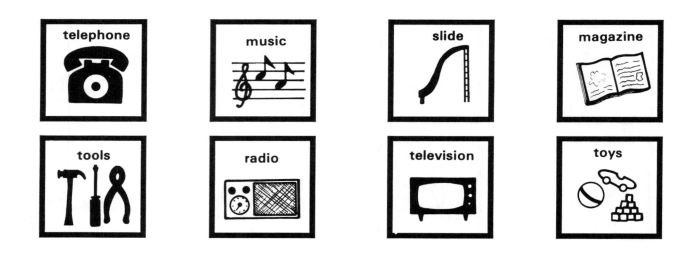

It's part of the playground.

You fix things with these. You build things with these.

Children play with these.

It's something you hear on the radio.

It rings. You call someone with this.

You turn it on to hear music.

You watch it. It plays movies and shows.

It's something you read.

Naming an Object

Directions: First review the symbols at the top of the page. The client chooses a symbol as each description is read.

Objective: After hearing a statement of an object's function and/or characteristics, the client will name the object.

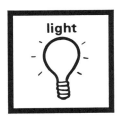

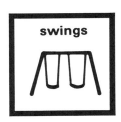
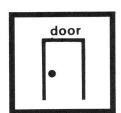

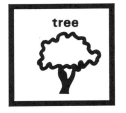
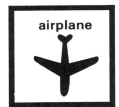

It's part of a room. You open it and shut it.

It flies. You ride it in the sky.

They're part of the playground.

You ride it in the water.

It's the opposite of dark.

It rides on a track.

You swim in this.

It grows outside. It has branches.

65

Naming an Object

Directions: First review the symbols at the top of the page. The client chooses a symbol as each description is read.

Objective: After hearing a statement of an object's function and/or characteristics, the client will name the object.

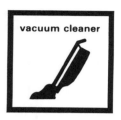
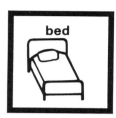

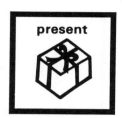
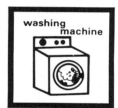
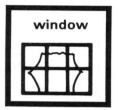
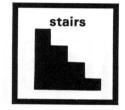
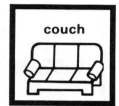

You get this on your birthday.

You put your head on this. It's on your bed.

It cleans the floor.

You look outside through this.

You sit on it. It has cushions.

It cleans your clothes.

You sleep in it. It has a pillow and a bedspread on it.

You climb these to go up and down.

Naming an Object

Directions: First review the symbols at the top of the page. The client chooses a symbol as each description is read.

Objective: After hearing a statement of an object's function and/or characteristics, the client will name the object.

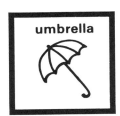
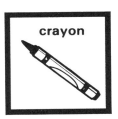
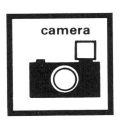
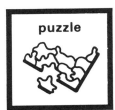

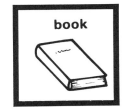
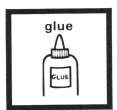

You take a picture with it. You put film in it.

It has pieces that you put together.

It's something you read. It has pages and a cover.

You color with it.

It keeps things stuck together.

You ring it.

It has keys. You type with it.

It keeps you dry in the rain.

Naming an Object/Person

Directions: First review the symbols at the top of the page. The client chooses a symbol as each description is read.

Objective: After hearing a statement of an object or person's function and/or characteristics, the client will name the object or person.

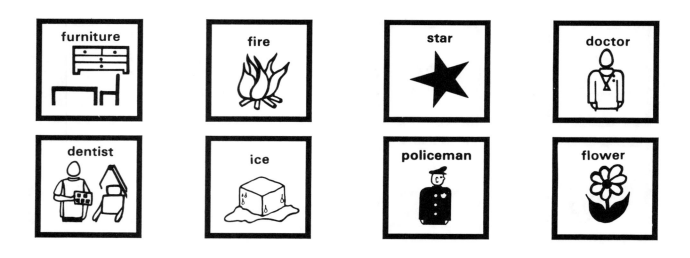

It grows. It has a stem.

It's hot. It burns.

It's someone you see when you're sick.

You put these things inside rooms. Bed, table and chairs are part of this group.

It's someone you call when you need help.

It's someone you see when you have a toothache.

It's cold. You put it in a cold drink.

You see this in the sky at night.

Naming a Setting

Directions: First review the symbols at the top of the page. The client chooses a symbol to name a place that matches each description as it is read. Try to read as few words as possible.

Objective: After hearing a list of words characteristic of a setting, the client will choose the appropriate setting.

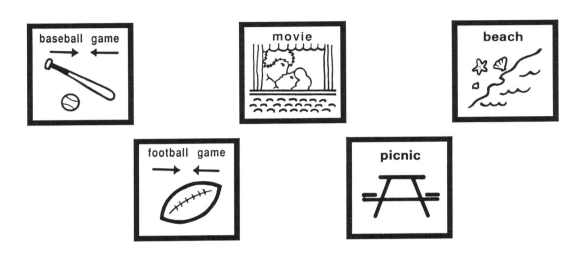

Where are you?

field - goal post - quarterback - 100 yard line - touchdown - field goal - helmet - half-time

sand - seashells - ocean - waves - sun bathers - surfers - pail and shovel - suntan lotion

large screen - stage - seats - tickets - popcorn - candy - usher - box office

diamond - bat - strike - homeplate - pitcher - homerun - catcher - glove - first base - triple play - innings

blanket - basket - thermos - cold food - paper plates

69

Naming a Setting

Directions: First review the symbols at the top of the page. The client chooses a symbol to name a place that matches each description as it is read. Try to read as few words as possible.

Objective: After hearing a list of words characteristic of a setting, the client will choose the appropriate setting.

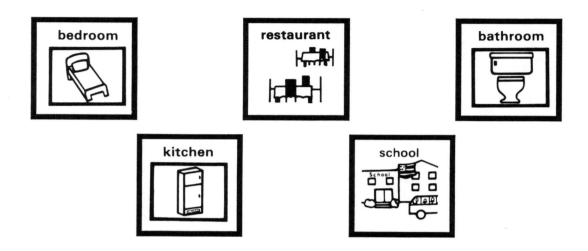

Where are you?

sink - towels - mirror - toothbrush - shower - toilet - bathtub

tables - chairs - cash register - booths - menu - waitress - salad bar - tip - chef - kitchen

dresser - closet - clothes - bed - lamp

desks - chairs - blackboard - students - classroom - teachers - books

sink - dishes - cabinets - silverware - can opener - refrigerator - stove - microwave oven - coffee pot - food

70

Naming a Setting

Directions: First review the symbols at the top of the page. The client chooses a symbol to name a place that matches each description as it is read. Try to read as few words as possible.

Objective: After hearing a list of words characteristic of a setting, the client will choose the appropriate setting.

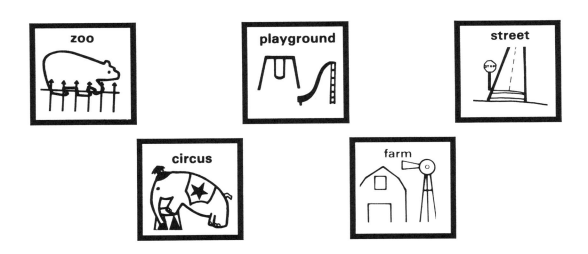

Where are you?

animals - cages - lions - tigers - monkeys - bears - zoo keeper

slide - swings - grass - sandbox - seesaw - merry-go-round - jungle gym

big tent - clowns - juggler - trapeze - ringmaster - seal - elephants - sword swallower - fire eater - tigers - hoops

animals - barn - pastures - tractor - cow - sheep - pig - chicken - horse - hay

curb - yellow line - corner - stop sign - pavement - speed limit - traffic light - dotted line - bus stop

Naming a Setting

Directions: First review the symbols at the top of the page. The client chooses a symbol to name a place that matches each description as it is read. Try to read as few words as possible.

Objective: After hearing a list of words characteristic of a setting, the client will choose the appropriate setting.

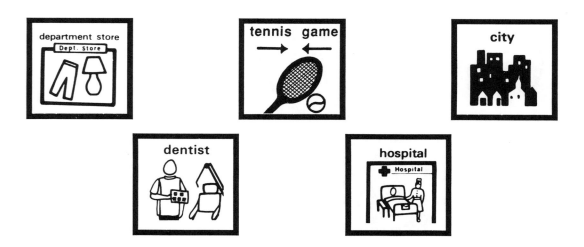

Where are you?

racquet - net - court - match - set

beds - nurses - patients - surgery - doctors - ambulance

merchandise - customers - sale - aisles - sales clerk - cash registers - dressing rooms

tall buildings - many people - heavy traffic - buses - sidewalks

chair - X-ray - fillings - patients - drill - novacaine

Naming a Setting

Directions: First review the symbols at the top of the page. The client chooses a symbol to name a place that matches each description as it is read. Try to read as few words as possible.

Objective: After hearing a list of words characteristic of a setting, the client will choose the appropriate setting.

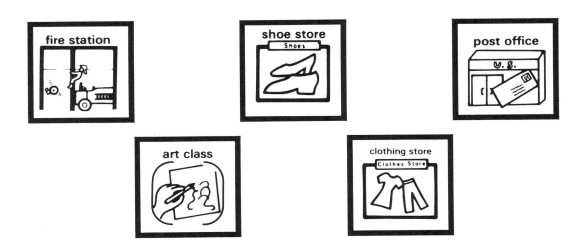

Where are you?

paper - crayons - scissors - glue - tissue paper - glitter - paint - paint brushes - clay

sneakers - shoes - boots - slippers - socks - shoe laces - sandals

fire engines - alarm - fire fighters - fire helmets - rain coats

shirts - pants - dresses - skirts - jeans - underwear - coats - blouses - jogging suits - ties - belts - suits - jackets - sweatshirts

stamps - mail boxes - postal clerk - packages - post cards

73

Naming a Setting

Directions: First review the symbols at the top of the page. The client chooses a symbol to name a place that matches each description as it is read. Try to read as few words as possible.

Objective: After hearing a list of words characteristic of a setting, the client will choose the appropriate setting.

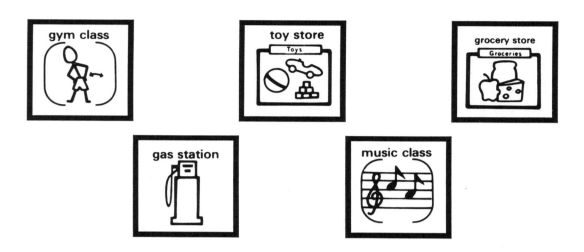

Where are you?

piano - bells - singing - tambourine - songs - triangle - drum
rhythm sticks - clapping

cars - fuel pumps - mechanics - oil - air pump -
gas attendant - tires

fruits - vegetables - meats - frozen foods - aisles -
cash registers - deli - eggs - fish - napkins - cheese -
peanut butter

mats - balls - exercise - running - basketball - balance beam
sports

games - dolls - trucks - computer games - puzzles - bikes -
roller skates - puppets - wagons - coloring books

Sentence Completion through Recall

Directions: First review the symbols at the top of the page. The client chooses a symbol to fill in the blank after each paragraph is read. One symbol will be left over and not used as an answer.

Objective: After comprehending the sentence, the client will recall the word to complete the sentence.

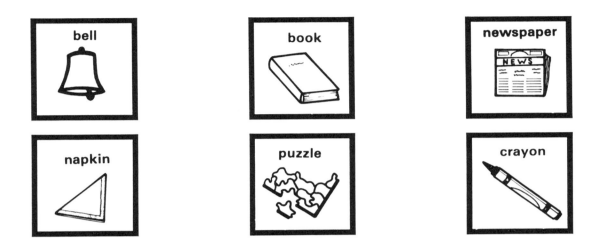

"Put your napkin on your lap. Oops, it fell on the floor. Pick up your _____."

"Did they deliver the morning newspaper yet? Every morning I like to read the _____."

"Here's a box of crayons. Color the sky with the blue _____."

"She rings the bell when it's time for dinner. Listen. I think I hear the _____."

"I'm missing too many puzzle pieces. How can I put together this _____?"

Sentence Completion through Recall

Directions: First review the symbols at the top of the page. The client chooses a symbol to fill in the blank after each paragraph is read. One symbol will be left over and not used as an answer.

Objective: After comprehending the sentence, the client will recall the word to complete the sentence.

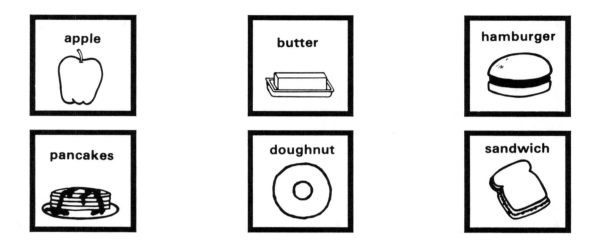

"One hamburger is not enough for me. I need another
_____."

"Here's a fresh batch of pancakes. Pour some syrup on your
_____."

"This popcorn doesn't taste buttery. We'd better put on
more melted _____."

"They bake the best doughnuts here. Waiter, I'll have a
jelly _____."

"Let's bake an apple pie. But first we'll go to the fruit stand
and buy some _____."

Sentence Completion through Recall

Directions: First review the symbols at the top of the page. The client chooses a symbol to fill in the blank after each paragraph is read. One symbol will be left over and not used as an answer.

Objective: After comprehending the sentence, the client will recall the word to complete the sentence.

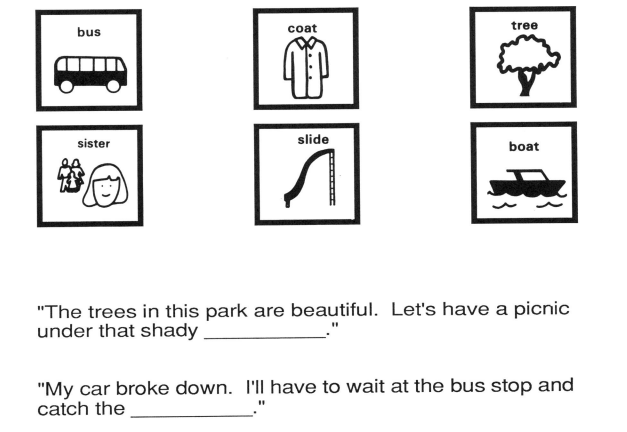

"The trees in this park are beautiful. Let's have a picnic under that shady _____."

"My car broke down. I'll have to wait at the bus stop and catch the _____."

"My brother loves to go down the slide at the playground. See, there he is on the _____."

"My sister knows what time the movie starts. Let's go home and ask my _____."

Sentence Completion through Recall

Directions: First review the symbols at the top of the page. The client chooses a symbol to fill in the blank after each paragraph is read. One symbol will be left over and not used as an answer.

Objective: After comprehending the sentence, the client will recall the word to complete the sentence.

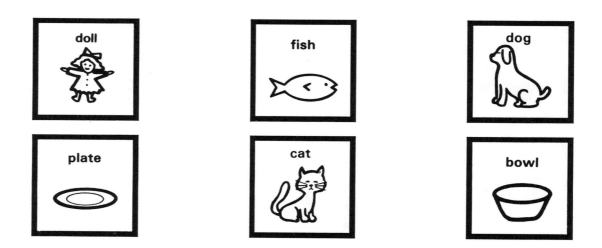

"My cat is sleeping on the chair. Oh no! The doorbell woke up my _____."

"I see you have a fish tank. May I look at the _____?"

"My baby sister wants a doll for her birthday. Let's go to the store and buy her a _____."

"Here's a spoon and a bowl. Pour the cereal in the _____."

"Our dogs should play together. My dog is in the backyard. Where is your _____?"

Sentence Completion through Recall

Directions: First review the symbols at the top of the page. The client chooses a symbol to fill in the blank after each paragraph is read. One symbol will be left over and not used as an answer.

Objective: After comprehending the sentence, the client will recall the word to complete the sentence.

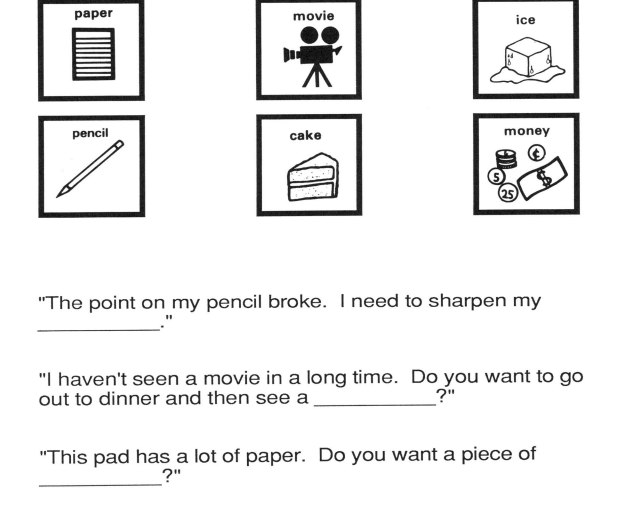

"The point on my pencil broke. I need to sharpen my _____."

"I haven't seen a movie in a long time. Do you want to go out to dinner and then see a _____?"

"This pad has a lot of paper. Do you want a piece of _____?"

"I don't have enough money to buy that book. Can you lend me some _____?"

"I put some ice cubes in my soda but it's still too warm. I need more _____."

Sentence Completion through Recall

Directions: First review the symbols at the top of the page. The client chooses a symbol to fill in the blank after each paragraph is read. One symbol will be left over and not used as an answer.

Objective: After comprehending the sentence, the client will recall the word to complete the sentence.

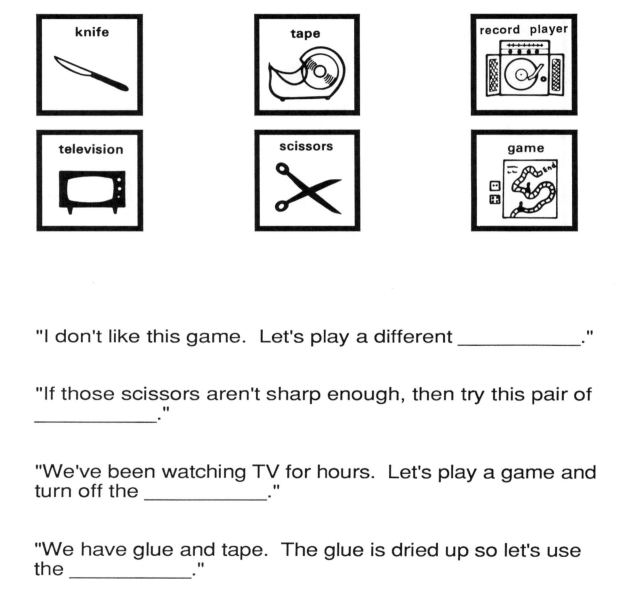

"I don't like this game. Let's play a different _____."

"If those scissors aren't sharp enough, then try this pair of _____."

"We've been watching TV for hours. Let's play a game and turn off the _____."

"We have glue and tape. The glue is dried up so let's use the _____."

"I bought a new record! I can't wait to play it on my _____."

Sentence Completion through Recall

Directions: First review the symbols at the top of the page. The client chooses a symbol to fill in the blank after each paragraph is read. One symbol will be left over and not used as an answer.

Objective: After comprehending the sentence, the client will recall the word to complete the sentence.

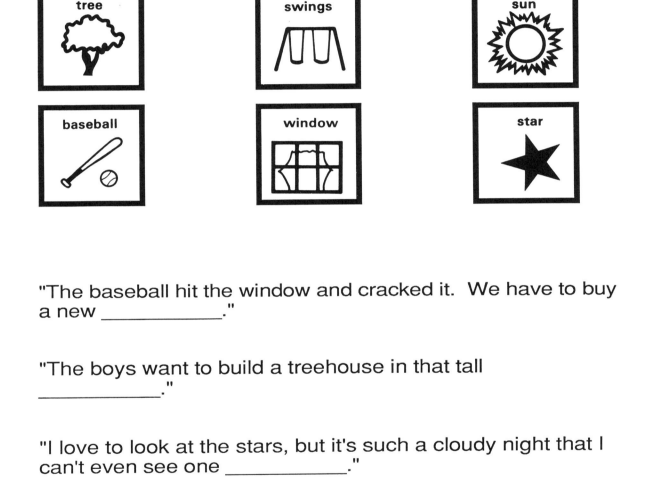

"The baseball hit the window and cracked it. We have to buy a new _____."

"The boys want to build a treehouse in that tall _____."

"I love to look at the stars, but it's such a cloudy night that I can't even see one _____."

" I like to play on the swings. Will someone please give me a push on the _____?"

"The kids are playing baseball outside. They need another player and asked if you know how to play _____."

Sentence Completion through Recall

Directions: First review the symbols at the top of the page. The client chooses a symbol to fill in the blank after each paragraph is read. One symbol will be left over and not used as an answer.

Objective: After comprehending the sentence, the client will recall the word to complete the sentence.

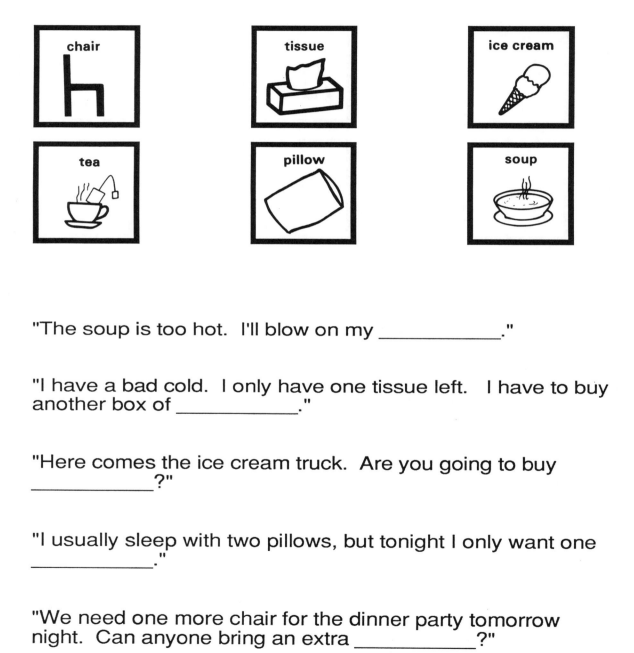

"The soup is too hot. I'll blow on my _____."

"I have a bad cold. I only have one tissue left. I have to buy another box of _____."

"Here comes the ice cream truck. Are you going to buy _____?"

"I usually sleep with two pillows, but tonight I only want one _____."

"We need one more chair for the dinner party tomorrow night. Can anyone bring an extra _____?"

Sentence Completion through Inference

Directions: First review the symbols at the top of the page. The client chooses a symbol to fill in the blank after each paragraph is read. One symbol will be left over and not used as an answer.

Objective: After comprehending the sentence, the client will infer the word to complete the sentence.

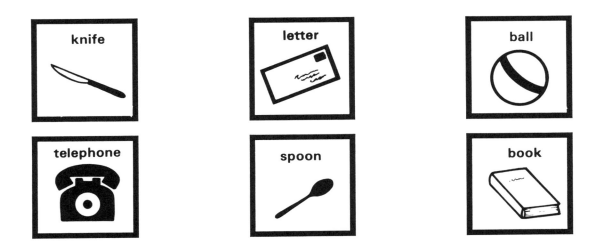

"I need to call home and talk to my mother. May I use your _____?"

"It's my turn to play. Throw the _____."

"Please stir the soup. Here's the _____."

"I can't wait to see what happens in the next chapter of this _____."

"Please cut the bread. Do you need to sharpen the _____?"

Sentence Completion through Inference

Directions: First review the symbols at the top of the page. The client chooses a symbol to fill in the blank after each paragraph is read. One symbol will be left over and not used as an answer.

Objective: After comprehending the sentence, the client will infer the word to complete the sentence.

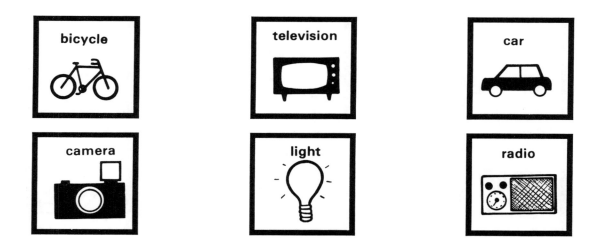

"We need to stop at the next gas station and get gas for the
_____."

"Let's hear the news and weather while we're driving. Turn
on the _____."

"Let's make the room quiet and dark for the surprise party.
Turn off the _____."

"I like to watch the news every night. Come with me and
we'll watch _____."

"I'll take your picture. Let me just put film in the
_____."

Sentence Completion through Inference

Directions: First review the symbols at the top of the page. The client chooses a symbol to fill in the blank after each paragraph is read. One symbol will be left over and not used as an answer.

Objective: After comprehending the sentence, the client will infer the word to complete the sentence.

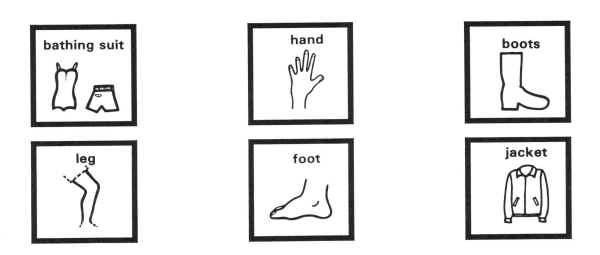

"You won't be warm enough in that shirt. You'd better wear a _____."

"We're going swimming at the beach. Don't forget to bring your _____."

"My new shoes hurt my _____."

"Don't wear your good shoes in the snow. Instead, put on your _____."

"Your pants ripped when you fell down. Did you cut your _____?"

Sentence Completion through Inference

Directions: First review the symbols at the top of the page. The client chooses a symbol to fill in the blank after each paragraph is read. One symbol will be left over and not used as an answer.

Objective: After comprehending the sentence, the client will infer the word to complete the sentence.

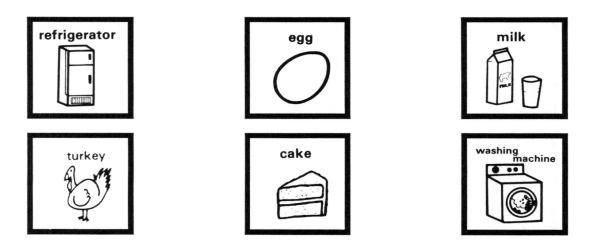

"Let's wash all the dirty clothes. Put the clothes in the
_____."

"At the farm we get to watch the chicken lay an
_____."

"I don't want any more milk. Please put it back in the
_____."

"The coffee is too hot. I need to put in more _____."

"It's your birthday. Blow out the candles on your
_____."

Sentence Completion through Inference

Directions: First review the symbols at the top of the page. The client chooses a symbol to fill in the blank after each paragraph is read. One symbol will be left over and not used as an answer.

Objective: After comprehending the sentence, the client will infer the word to complete the sentence.

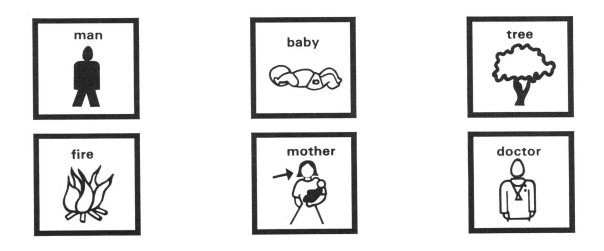

"I'm meeting my parents at the airport. Look! There's my father and _____."

"I have a new little brother because my mother had a _____."

"Call the fire department. I see a _____."

"Last night, lightning struck the branch of that _____."

"You look very sick. You'd better go to the _____."

Sentence Completion through Inference

Directions: First review the symbols at the top of the page. The client chooses a symbol to fill in the blank after each paragraph is read. One symbol will be left over and not used as an answer.

Objective: After comprehending the sentence, the client will infer the word to complete the sentence.

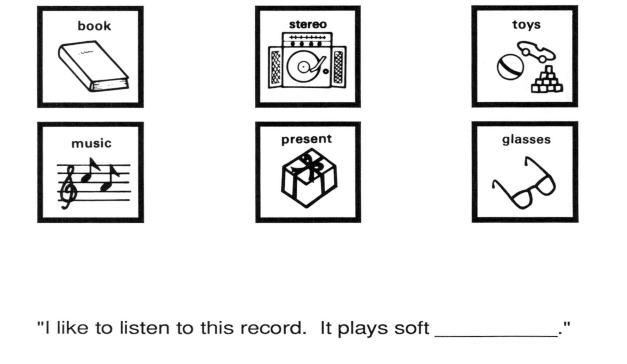

"I like to listen to this record. It plays soft _____."

"I want to read the magazine, but I can't see it clearly. I need to put on my _____."

"What a great movie! Now I want to read the _____!"

"It's your birthday. Hurry and open your _____."

"Jonathon is a good baby. He never gets tired of playing with his _____."

Sentence Completion through Inference

Directions: First review the symbols at the top of the page. The client chooses a symbol to fill in the blank after each paragraph is read. One symbol will be left over and not used as an answer.

Objective: After comprehending the sentence, the client will infer the word to complete the sentence.

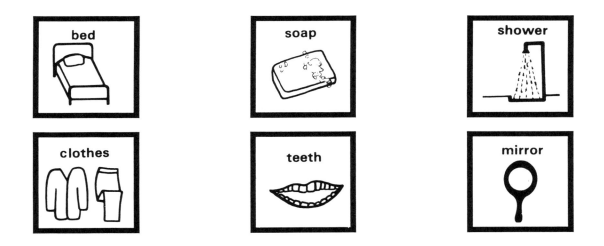

"It's time to do the laundry. Give me your dirty
_____."

"I can still taste that pizza. I'll go brush my _____."

"I'm dirty all over. I need to take a _____."

"Take a look at yourself. In the bathroom there's a
_____."

"I'm tired. It's time for me to go to _____."

Sentence Completion through Inference

Directions: First review the symbols at the top of the page. The client chooses a symbol to fill in the blank after each paragraph is read. One symbol will be left over and not used as an answer.

Objective: After comprehending the sentence, the client will infer the word to complete the sentence.

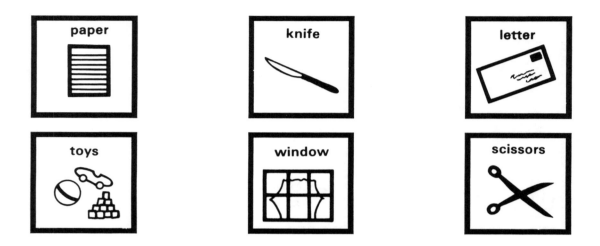

"There's a nice breeze outside. Let's feel it inside the house. Open the _____."

"Please help cut out these heart shapes. Here's a pair of _____."

"What time does the mailman come? I want to mail this _____."

"On their birthdays we buy children new _____."

"I want to draw a picture. I need another sheet of _____."

Sentence Completion through Inference

Directions: First review the symbols at the top of the page. The client chooses a symbol to fill in the blank after each paragraph is read. One symbol will be left over and not used as an answer.

Objective: After comprehending the sentence, the client will infer the word to complete the sentence.

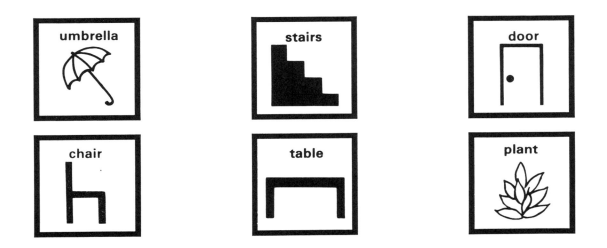

"My bedroom isn't down here. I have to go up the _____."

"It's time for dinner. Please help me set the _____."

"We're going to get wet out here in the rain. Open the _____."

"The TV in the other room is too loud. Please shut my bedroom _____."

"Please watch my house while I'm gone. Don't forget to feed my cat and water my _____."

Sentence Completion through Inference

Directions: First review the symbols at the top of the page. The client chooses a symbol to fill in the blank after each paragraph is read. One symbol will be left over and not used as an answer.

Objective: After comprehending the sentence, the client will infer the word to complete the sentence.

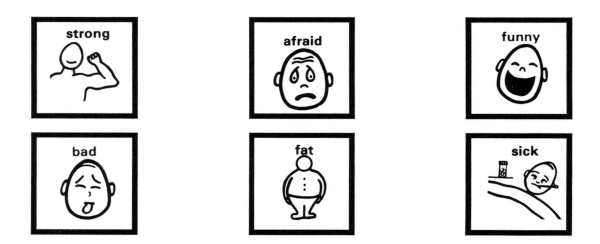

"Whenever we watch scary movies I feel _____."

"I can't stop laughing because that joke is very _____."

"This fever makes me feel _____."

"Do your exercises and be _____."

"Those rotten tomatoes taste _____."

Sentence Completion in a Paragraph

Directions: First review the symbols at the top of the page. The client chooses a symbol to fill in the blank as the story is read.

Objective: After comprehending the sentence in the context of a paragraph, the client will infer the word to complete the sentence.

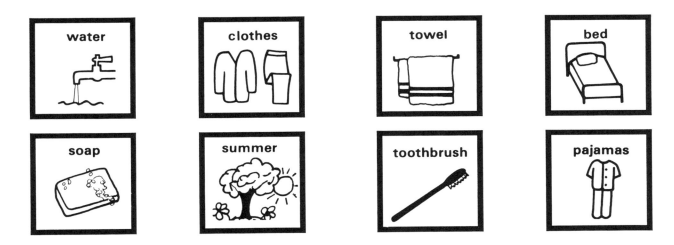

A Silly Morning

Scott woke up early and jumped out of _____. He went into the bathroom to brush his teeth. He took out the toothpaste but he couldn't find his _____. Then he saw it on the sink.

After he brushed his teeth, Scott started to wash his face. He turned on the _____ and made lots of bubbles with the _____. Then he dried his face with a _____.

It was a nice day and Scott couldn't wait to go outside. He opened the door and stepped outside. Suddenly, Scott looked down at his feet and saw his slippers! Then he looked at his body. He was so excited about going outside that he had forgotten to take off his _____ and put on his _____.

93

Sentence Completion in a Paragraph

Directions: First review the symbols at the top of the page. The client chooses a symbol to fill in the blank as the story is read.

Objective: After comprehending the sentence in the context of a paragraph, the client will infer the word to complete the sentence.

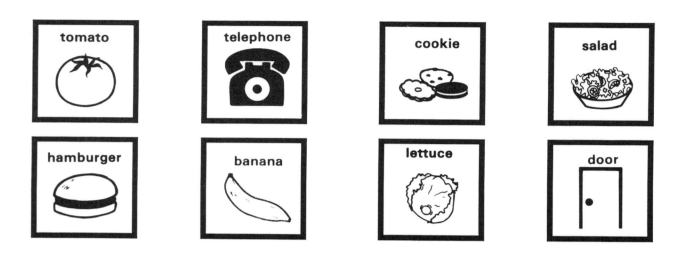

The Mixed-up Salad

Mary had invited friends to her house for a picnic. She started the barbecue to cook hot dogs and _____. Next she took out a big bowl to make a salad. Green vegetables were needed for the salad, so she put in cucumbers and _____. Then she sliced ripe red _____ and some carrots. For the dessert, Mary baked some delicious chocolate chip _____.

Mary heard the doorbell and went to answer the _____. It was Charles. "I'm not good at cooking, but can I help you make anything?" he asked.

"Sure," said Mary. "The fruit cups are easy to make. Just peel this _____ and then slice it. After you finish that, put the banana pieces in the little cups."

"Okay," said Charles, and he started peeling the banana.

A few minutes later Mary looked over at Charles. She saw little pieces of banana mixed in with tomatoes and lettuce. "Charles," she laughed. "You aren't very good at cooking. You put the bananas in the _____!"

94

Sentence Completion in a Paragraph

Directions: First review the symbols at the top of the page. The client chooses a symbol to fill in the blank as the story is read.

Objective: After comprehending the sentence in the context of a paragraph, the client will infer the word to complete the sentence.

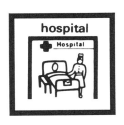

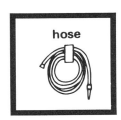

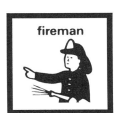

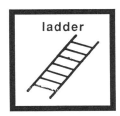

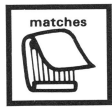

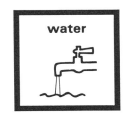

Look Out for Flying Water!

Our school had a visitor today for Fire Prevention Week. His name is Paul and he is a _____. He came riding to school in his red _____. Paul greeted everyone and then talked about the fire truck. He climbed up high on the _____. He told us that the ladder helps him reach high buildings.

When Paul climbed down from the fire truck he asked, "What is used to spray water on the fires?" We all told him that the firemen use the long _____. "Yes," said Paul, "and this big hose can spray the _____ hard and fast."

Then Paul told us how dangerous fires can be. If people get burned in a fire, an ambulance takes them to a _____. Paul told us that we can prevent fires by not playing with _____. He lit a match to show us the flame. Someone immediately threw a glass of _____ at Paul! It put out the _____, but it sure made Paul wet.

95

Sentence Completion in a Paragraph

Directions: First review the symbols at the top of the page. The client chooses a symbol to fill in the blank as the story is read.

Objective: After comprehending the sentence in the context of a paragraph, the client will infer the word to complete the sentence.

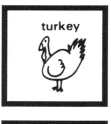
turkey

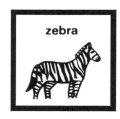
zebra

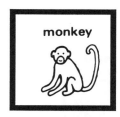
monkey

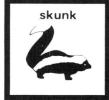
skunk

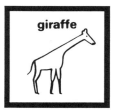
giraffe

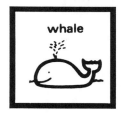
whale

The Zoo Game

"What should we do today?" Mark asked Jackie.

"Hmmm," Jackie thought out loud. "Let's go to the zoo. When we get there, let's play a guessing game. We'll describe the animals to each other and guess what they are."

"Okay," Mark said. "Let's go!"

When they arrived at the zoo, Mark said, "Close your eyes. This cage has an animal with stripes all around its body. What is it?"

"It sounds like a _____," Jackie said.

They walked a little further. "The animal in this cage has a stripe only on its tail," said Jackie. "And it can sure be smelly!"

"Then it must be a _____," laughed Mark.

As they walked along Mark said, "This animal is swinging from a branch by its tail. I bet it would love a banana."

"I guess it's a _____," said Jackie.

At the next enclosure she said, "This animal has a neck longer than any other animal at the zoo."

"A long neck?" Mark repeated. "It sounds like a _____."

While they were walking to the next cage Mark said, "I'm thinking of an animal that lives in the ocean. It is very large and spouts water out near the top of its head."

"Hmmm," thought Jackie. "A seal is small and a shark doesn't spout water. It must be a _____."

In front of the last cage Jackie said, "This is a big bird that does not like Thanksgiving."

"That can only be a _____," Mark laughed.

Both children agreed it had been an especially fun day at the zoo.

Determining the Referent

Directions: First review the symbols at the top of the page. As you read each paragraph, emphasize the underlined word. The client chooses a symbol to substitute for the underlined word after each question is asked. Use the first one as an example. When the client chooses an answer, read the sentence aloud, re-placing the underlined word with the client's answer.

Objective: After hearing a sentence using nouns, the client will state the noun replaced by the under-lined referent.

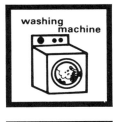

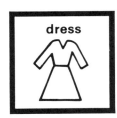

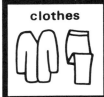

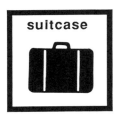

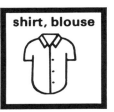

I just put my clothes in the washing machine. **<u>It</u>** will proba-bly run for half an hour. (What does the word "it" stand for?)

I'll wear my red dress to the party. When is **<u>it</u>**? (What does the word "it" stand for?)

I need new clothes for the party. I'll buy **them** next week. (What does the word "them" stand for?)

I bought Steve a shirt for his birthday. I hope he likes **<u>it</u>**. (What does the word "it" stand for?)

I'll pack my dress in the suitcase. I want to wear **<u>it</u>** on my trip. (What does the word "it" stand for?)

Determining the Referent

Directions: First review the symbols at the top of the page. As you read each paragraph, emphasize the underlined word. The client chooses a symbol to substitute for the underlined word after each question is asked. Use the first one as an example. When the client chooses an answer, read the sentence aloud, replacing the underlined word with the client's answer.

Objective: After hearing a sentence using nouns, the client will state the noun replaced by the underlined referent.

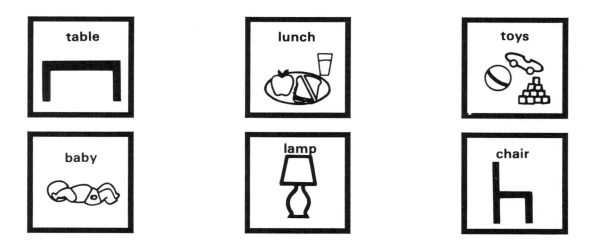

I put the lamp near the edge of the table. I hope **it** doesn't fall. (What does the word "it" stand for?)

The baby keeps crawling into the chair. I'll have to move **it**. (What does the word "it" stand for?)

The baby is playing and doesn't want to eat lunch now. Maybe he'll have **it** later. (What does the word "it" stand for?)

We're going to eat lunch on this table. Everyone pull your chair closer to **it**. (What does the word "it" stand for?)

Here's a new toy for the baby. Give **it** to **him**. (What does the word "it" stand for? What does the word "him" stand for?)

There's a fly on the lamp. I hope **it** doesn't break when I'm swatting. (What does the word "it" stand for?)

Determining the Referent

Directions: First review the symbols at the top of the page. As you read each paragraph, emphasize the underlined word. The client chooses a symbol to substitute for the underlined word after each question is asked. Use the first one as an example. When the client chooses an answer, read the sentence aloud, replacing the underlined word with the client's answer.

Objective: After hearing a sentence using nouns, the client will state the noun replaced by the underlined referent.

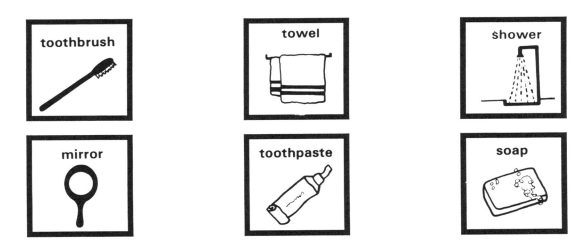

This towel is too wet for me to use after my shower. I'll take another **one**. (What does the word "one" stand for?)

The toothpaste squirted all over the mirror. I'll have to wipe **it** until it shines. (What does the word "it" stand for?)

The toothbrushes on this shelf come in many colors. Which **one** do you want to buy? (What does the word "one" stand for?)

I dropped the soap on the floor. Don't step on **it**. (What does the word "it" stand for?)

I have a toothbrush but there's not enough toothpaste. I'll have to get **some** at the store. (What does the word "some" stand for?)

We need more soap in the shower. Put this bar of soap in **there**. (What does the word "there" stand for?)

Determining the Referent

Directions: First review the symbols at the top of the page. As you read each paragraph, emphasize the underlined word. The client chooses a symbol to substitute for the underlined word after each question is asked. Use the first one as an example. When the client chooses an answer, read the sentence aloud, replacing the underlined word with the client's answer.

Objective: After hearing a sentence using nouns, the client will state the noun replaced by the underlined referent.

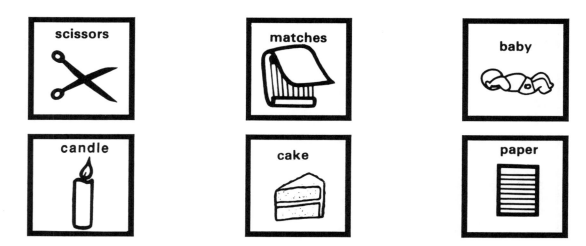

I tried to light the candle but the match went out. Do you have another **one**? (What does the word "one" stand for?)

Cut the paper in half. Now **it** is just the right size. (What does the word "it" stand for?)

The scissors are on the desk. Can you reach **them**? (What does the word "them" stand for?)

We told the baby not to play with matches. We hope **she** listens. (What does the word "she" stand for?)

Blow out the candles on your cake. Look, there is still **one** left. (What does the word "one" stand for?)

Cut the cake into two pieces. Now we can both have **some**. (What does the word "some" stand for?)

Determining the Referent

Directions: First review the symbols at the top of the page. As you read each paragraph, emphasize the underlined word. The client chooses a symbol to substitute for the underlined word after each question is asked. Use the first one as an example. When the client chooses an answer, read the sentence aloud, replacing the underlined word with the client's answer.

Objective: After hearing a sentence using nouns, the client will state the noun replaced by the underlined referent.

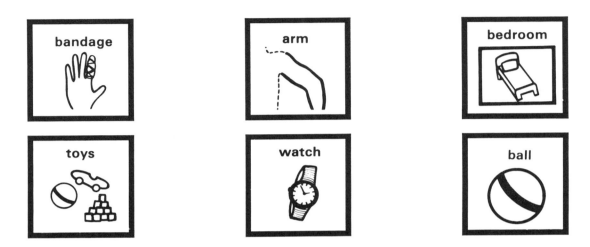

My watch hurts my arm. I'll have to put a bandage on **it**. (What does the word "it" stand for?)

I have many toys but I like my ball the best. **It** is my favorite. (What does the word "it" stand for?)

My bedroom is a mess because toys are all over. I have to clean **it**. (What does the word "it" stand for?)

I lost my watch in the bedroom. I hope I can find **it**. (What does the word "it" stand for?)

I'll put all of my toys in the closet. But first, I'll put **them** in a pile. (What does the word "them" stand for?)

This bandage isn't big enough for my arm. I'll need a bigger **one**. (What does the word "one" stand for?)

Determining the Referent

Directions: First review the symbols at the top of the page. As you read each paragraph, emphasize the underlined word. The client chooses a symbol to substitute for the underlined word after each question is asked. Use the first one as an example. When the client chooses an answer, read the sentence aloud, replacing the underlined word with the client's answer.

Objective: After hearing a sentence using nouns, the client will state the noun replaced by the underlined referent.

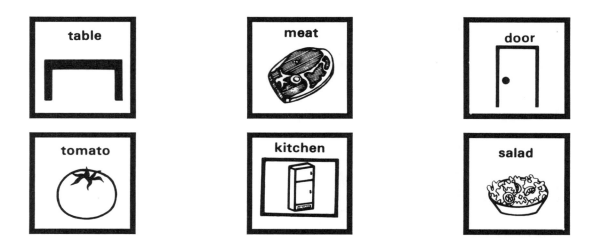

I put more tomatoes in the salad. Do you want to mix **it**? (What does the word "it" stand for?)

I put the salad on the table but the meat is still in the kitchen. Would you please get **it**? (What does the word "it" stand for?)

The table is too close to the door. Let's move **it**. (What does the word "it" stand for?)

I opened the kitchen door but it won't stay open. Will you try to make **it** stay open? (What does the word "it" stand for?)

The dinner is good but I didn't get a tomato. Please pass **one** to me. (What does the word "one" stand for?)

The kitchen gets too hot when we cook meat. Let's open the door and cool **it** off. (What does the word "it" stand for?)

Determining the Referent

Directions: First review the symbols at the top of the page. As you read each paragraph, emphasize the underlined word. The client chooses a symbol to substitute for the underlined word after each question is asked. Use the first one as an example. When the client chooses an answer, read the sentence aloud, replacing the underlined word with the client's answer.

Objective: After hearing a sentence using nouns, the client will state the noun replaced by the underlined referent.

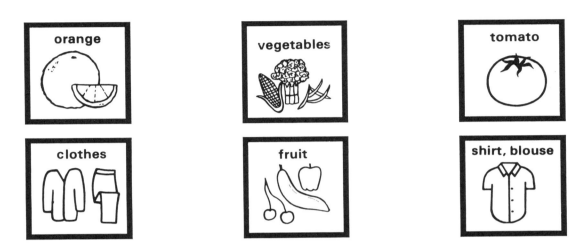

I think I'll eat a tomato instead of an orange. Here's **one** for you too. (What does the word "one" stand for?)

The vegetables are a little bit dirty. We should wash **them**. (What does the word "them" stand for?)

I ripped my shirt and had to buy all new clothes. I'll hang **them** up in the closet. (What does the word "them" stand for?)

All of the fruits are in the bowl except an orange. Can you get **one**? (What does the word "one" stand for?)

The tomato stained my shirt. I hope the stain is gone after I wash **it**. (What does the word "it" stand for?)

Our trees grow three different kinds of fruit. Let's see if **they** are ripe enough to pick. (What does the word "they" stand for?)

Body Part-Action Association

Directions: First review the symbols at the top of the page. The client chooses a symbol to fill in the blank as the sentence is read. Some sentences may have more than one answer.

Objective: The client will choose the actions most commonly performed by the given body part.

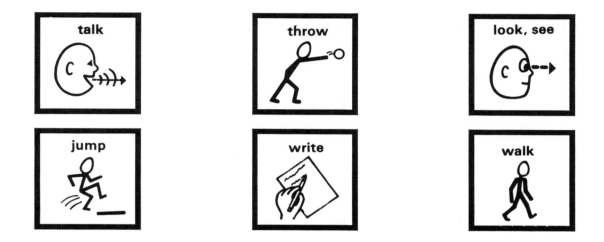

Your eyes help you _____.

Your legs help you _____.

Your mouth helps you _____.

Your arms help you _____.

Your feet help you _____.

Your hands help you _____.

Body Part-Action Association

Directions: First review the symbols at the top of the page. The client chooses a symbol to fill in the blank as the sentence is read. Some sentences may have more than one answer.

Objective: The client will choose the actions most commonly performed by the given body part.

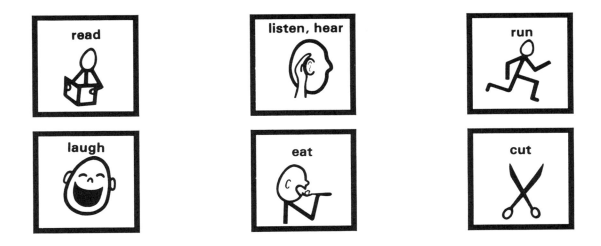

Your legs help you _____.

Your ears help you _____.

Your eyes help you _____.

Your feet help you _____.

Your hands help you _____.

Your mouth helps you _____.

Action-Body Part Association

Directions: First review the symbols at the top of the page. The client chooses a symbol to fill in the blank as the sentence is read. Some sentences may have more than one correct answer. There may be one symbol left over and not used as an answer.

Objective: The client will choose the body parts most commonly used to complete the given action.

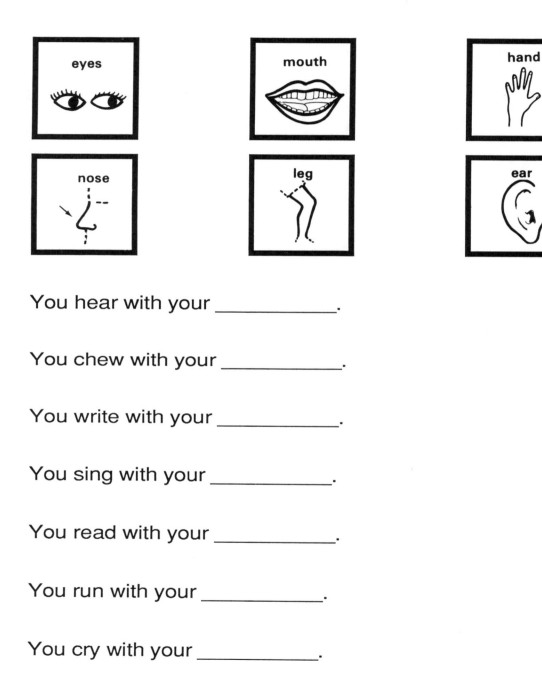

You hear with your _____.

You chew with your _____.

You write with your _____.

You sing with your _____.

You read with your _____.

You run with your _____.

You cry with your _____.

Action-Body Part Association

Directions: First review the symbols at the top of the page. The client chooses a symbol to fill in the blank as the sentence is read. Some sentences may have more than one correct answer. There may be one symbol left over and not used as an answer.

Objective: The client will choose the body parts most commonly used to complete the given action.

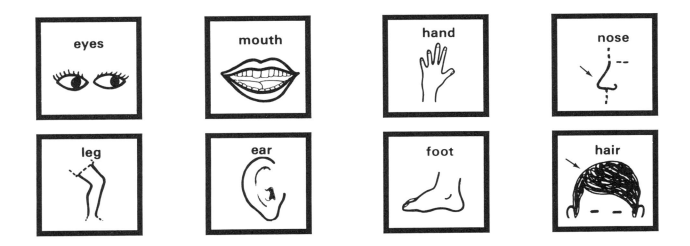

You catch with your _____.

You smell with your _____.

You eat with your _____.

You kick with your _____.

You listen with your _____.

You smile with your _____.

You walk with your _____.

You draw with your _____.

Action-Body Part Association

Directions: First review the symbols at the top of the page. The client chooses a symbol to fill in the blank as the sentence is read. Some sentences may have more than one correct answer. There may be one symbol left over and not used as an answer.

Objective: The client will choose the body parts most commonly used to complete the given action.

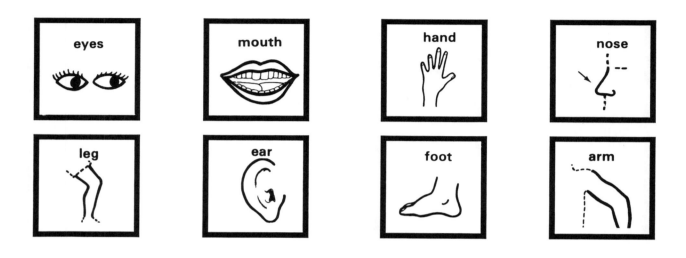

You jump with your _____.

You breathe with your _____.

You talk with your _____.

You swim with your _____.

You throw with your _____.

You see with your _____.

You type with your _____.

108

Baby Animal Association

Directions: First review the symbols at the top of the page. The client then chooses a symbol to fill in the blank as the sentence is read. One symbol will be left over and not used as an answer.

Objective: The client will choose the animal associated with the baby of that animal.

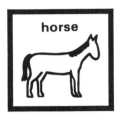
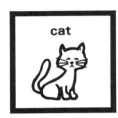
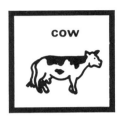
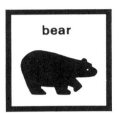

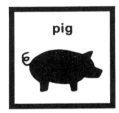
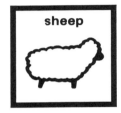
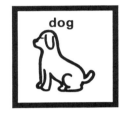
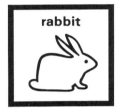

A puppy is a baby _____.

A lamb is a baby _____.

A cub is a baby _____.

A kitten is a baby _____.

A calf is a baby _____.

A piglet is a baby _____.

A colt is a baby _____.

Associating Objects with Locations

Directions: First review the symbols at the top of the page. Explain that rooms are symbolized by a box around an important appliance or piece of furniture from that room (point to an example). Without the box, the symbol represents just the appliance or furniture. The client chooses a symbol to name a location as each question is read. Some questions may have more than one correct answer. One symbol will be left over and not used as an answer.

Objective: The client will choose all of the locations where a given object may be found.

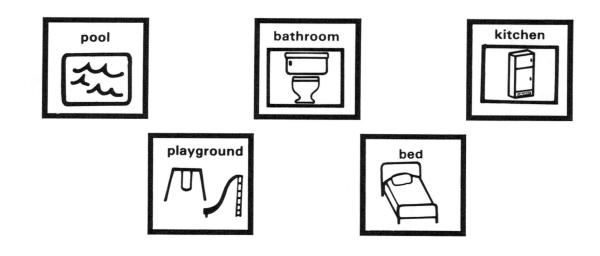

Where would you find _____?

table

blanket

bathtub

swings

bowl

shampoo

Associating Objects with Locations

Directions: First review the symbols at the top of the page. The client chooses a symbol to name a location as each question is read. Some questions may have more than one correct answer. One symbol will be left over and not used as an answer.

Objective: The client will choose all of the locations where a given object may be found.

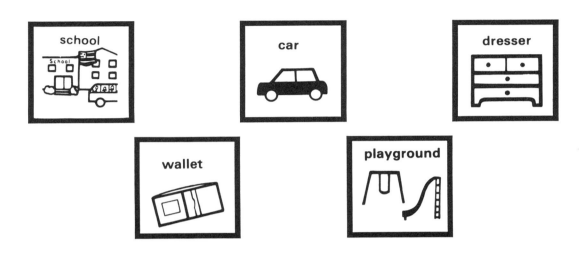

Where would you find _____?

chalkboard

money

wheels

books

socks

trunk

111

Associating Objects with Locations

Directions: First review the symbols at the top of the page. The client chooses a symbol to name a location as each question is read. Some questions may have more than one correct answer. One symbol will be left over and not used as an answer.

Objective: The client will choose all of the locations where a given object may be found.

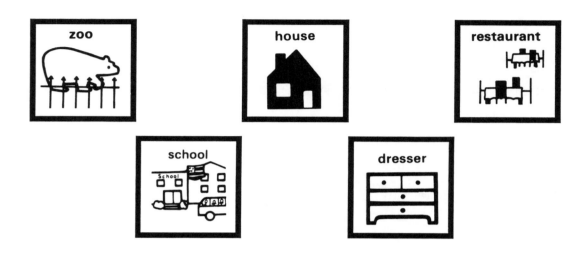

Where would you find _____?

cash register

monkeys

bedroom

pajamas

giraffes

menu

112

Associating Objects with Locations

Directions: First review the symbols at the top of the page. Explain that rooms are symbolized by a box around an important appliance or piece of furniture from that room (point to an example). Without the box, the symbol represents just the appliance or furniture. The client chooses a symbol to name a location as each question is read. Some questions may have more than one correct answer. One symbol will be left over and not used as an answer.

Objective: The client will choose all of the locations where a given object may be found.

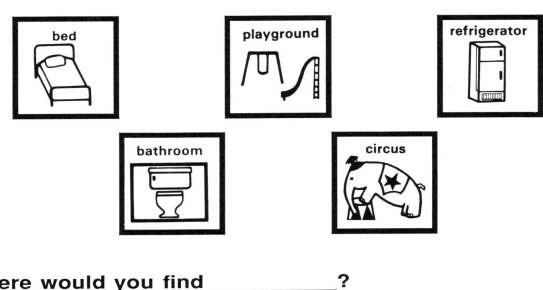

Where would you find _____?

slide

pillow

cheese

toothpaste

sandbox

juice

Associating Objects with Locations

Directions: First review the symbols at the top of the page. The client chooses a symbol to name a location as each question is read. Some questions may have more than one correct answer. One symbol will be left over and not used as an answer.

Objective: The client will choose all of the locations where a given object may be found.

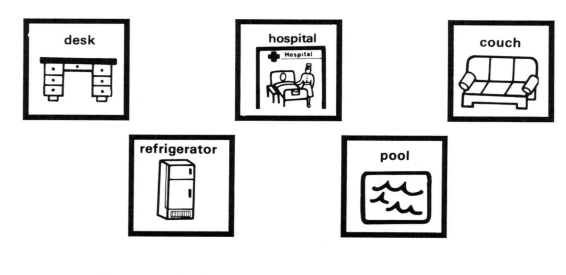

Where would you find _____?

typewriter

lamp

doctor

milk

nurse

water

Associating Objects with Locations

Directions: First review the symbols at the top of the page. Explain that rooms are symbolized by a box around an important appliance or piece of furniture from that room (point to an example). Without the box, the symbol represents just the appliance or furniture. The client chooses a symbol to name a location as each question is read. Some questions may have more than one correct answer. One symbol will be left over and not used as an answer.

Objective: The client will choose all of the locations where a given object may be found.

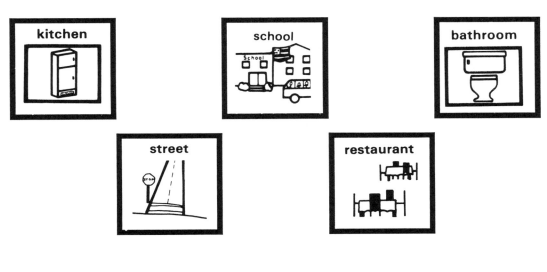

Where would you find _____?

towel

table

sink

window

toilet

chalkboard

115

Associating Locations with Objects

Directions: First review the symbols at the top of the page. The client chooses a symbol to name an item found in a specific location as each question is read. Some questions may have more than one correct answer. One symbol may be left over and not used as an answer.

Objective: The client will choose all of the objects that may be found in a given location.

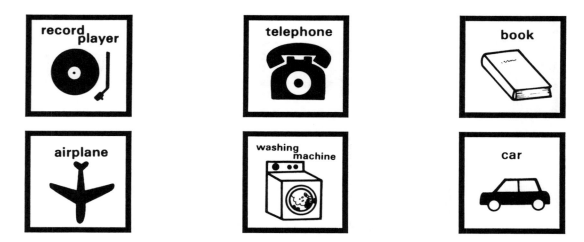

What would you find in/on a _____?

shelf

library

laundramat

parking lot

street

airport

Associating Locations with Objects

Directions: First review the symbols at the top of the page. The client chooses a symbol to name an item found in a specific location as each question is read. Some questions may have more than one correct answer. One symbol may be left over and not used as an answer.

Objective: The client will choose all of the objects that may be found in a given location.

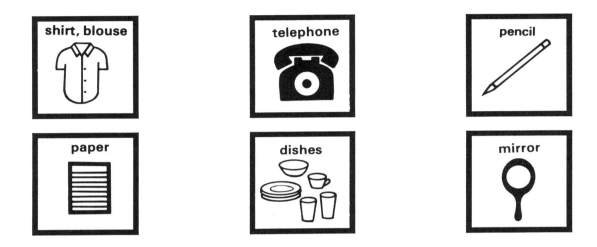

What would you find in/on a _____?

desk

kitchen

restaurant

clothes store

school

dresser

Associating Locations with Objects

Directions: First review the symbols at the top of the page. The client chooses a symbol to name an item found in a specific location as each question is read. Some questions may have more than one correct answer. One symbol may be left over and not used as an answer.

Objective: The client will choose all of the objects that may be found in a given location.

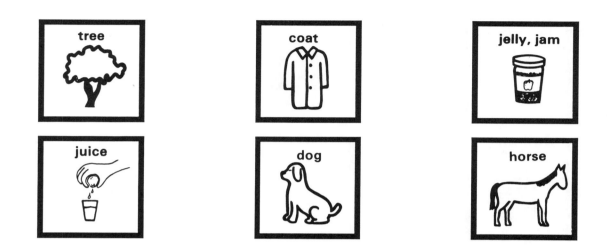

What would you find in/on a _____?

refrigerator

closet

jar

pet shop

hanger

farm

118

Associating Locations with Objects

Directions: First review the symbols at the top of the page. The client chooses a symbol to name an item found in a specific location as each question is read. Some questions may have more than one correct answer. One symbol may be left over and not used as an answer.

Objective: The client will choose all of the objects that may be found in a given location.

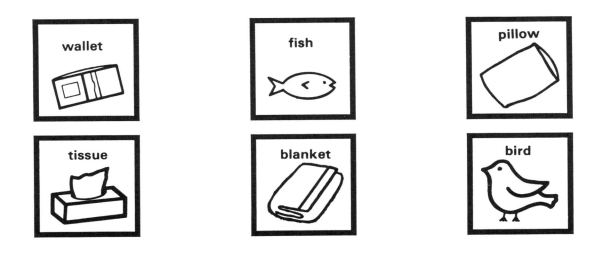

What would you find in/on a _____?

bed

cage

pocket

bathroom

purse

couch

119

Associating Locations with Objects

Directions: First review the symbols at the top of the page. The client chooses a symbol to name an item found in a specific location as each question is read. Some questions may have more than one correct answer. One symbol may be left over and not used as an answer.

Objective: The client will choose all of the objects that may be found in a given location.

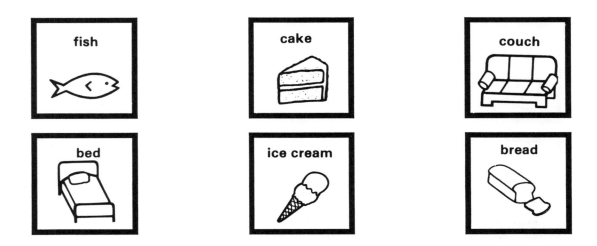

What would you find in/on a _____?

bakery

sandwich

freezer

furniture store

bedroom

fish bowl

Associating Locations with Objects

Directions: First review the symbols at the top of the page. The client chooses a symbol to name an item found in a specific location as each question is read. Some questions may have more than one correct answer. One symbol may be left over and not used as an answer.

Objective: The client will choose all of the objects that may be found in a given location.

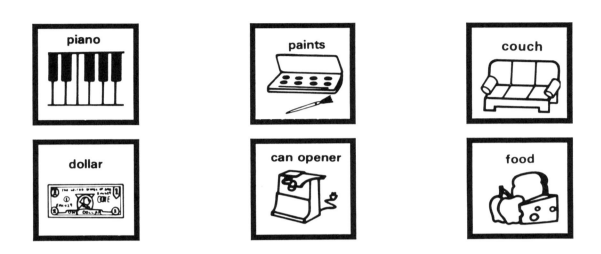

What would you find in/at a _____?

art class

kitchen

bank

music class

restaurant

living room

Associating Locations with Objects

Directions: First review the symbols at the top of the page. The client chooses a symbol to name an item found in a specific location as each question is read. Some questions may have more than one correct answer. One symbol may be left over and not used as an answer.

Objective: The client will choose all of the objects that may be found in a given location.

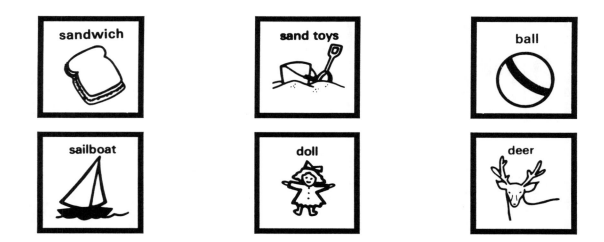

What would you find in/at a _____?

dollhouse

gym class

beach

forest

lunch box

lake

What Questions

Directions: First review the symbols at the top of the page. The client chooses a symbol as each question is read. One or more symbols will be left over and not used as answers.

Objective: The client will choose the animal associated with the sound presented in the question.

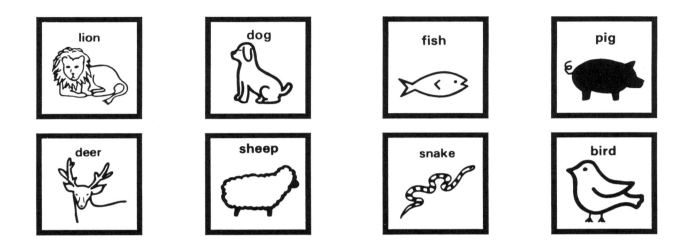

What oinks?

What baas?

What roars?

What barks?

What hisses?

What chirps?

123

What Questions

Directions: First review the symbols at the top of the page. The client chooses a symbol as each question is read. One or more symbols will be left over and not used as answers.

Objective: The client will choose the animal associated with the sound presented in the question.

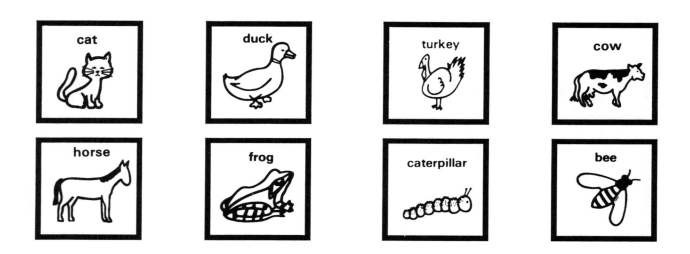

What moos?

What gobbles?

What quacks?

What neighs?

What meows?

What croaks?

What buzzes?

124

What Questions

Directions: First review the symbols at the top of the page. The client chooses a symbol as each question is read. Some questions may have more than one correct answer.

Objective: The client will choose the item (s) commonly associated with the action presented in the question.

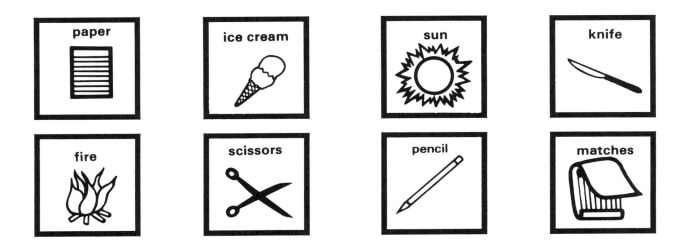

What writes?

What burns?

What cuts?

What rips?

What melts?

What shines?

What Questions

Directions: First review the symbols at the top of the page. The client chooses a symbol as each question is read. Some questions may have more than one correct answer.

Objective: The client will choose the item (s) commonly associated with the action presented in the question.

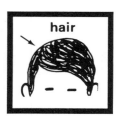
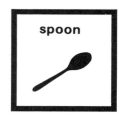
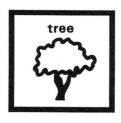
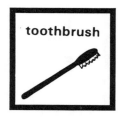

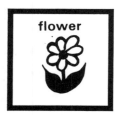
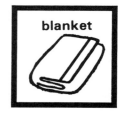
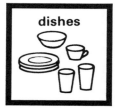

What stirs?

What blooms?

What brushes?

What folds?

What grows?

What breaks?

What Questions

Directions: First review the symbols at the top of the page. The client chooses a symbol as each question is read. Some questions may have more than one correct answer.

Objective: The client will choose the item (s) commonly associated with the action presented in the question.

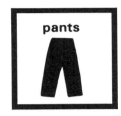
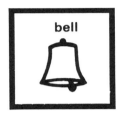
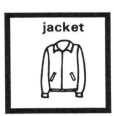
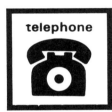
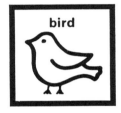
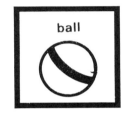
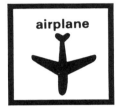

What bounces?

What rings?

What flies?

What drives?

What zips?

What rolls?

What Questions

Directions: First review the symbols at the top of the page. The client chooses a symbol as each question is read. Some questions may have more than one correct answer.

Objective: The client will choose the item (s) commonly associated with the action presented in the question.

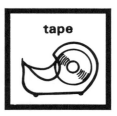

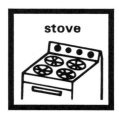

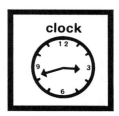

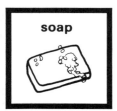

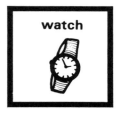

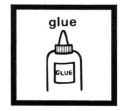

What sticks?

What cleans?

What ticks?

What swims?

What cooks?

What Questions

Directions: First review the symbols at the top of the page. The client chooses a symbol as each question is read. Some questions may have more than one correct answer.

Objective: The client will choose the item (s) commonly associated with the action presented in the question.

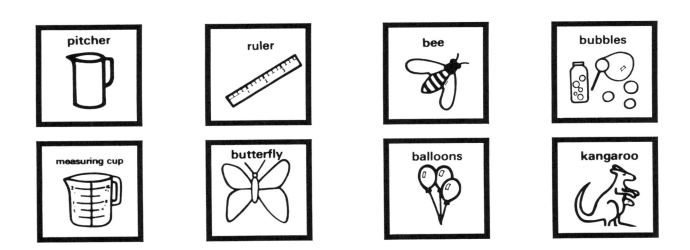

What flies?

What pours?

What pops?

What stings?

What measures?

What hops?

129

Object Association

Directions: First review the symbols at the top of the page. The client chooses a symbol that goes with the given item as each question is read. One symbol will be left over and not used as an answer.

Objective: The client will choose an object associated with a given object.

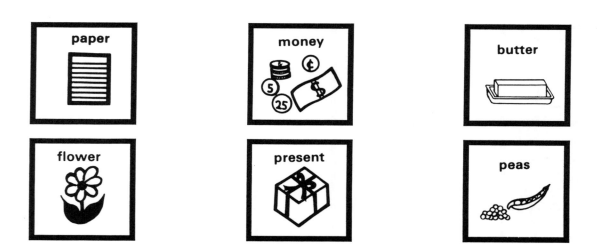

What goes with _____?

water

bread

cash register

party

pencil

Object Association

Directions: First review the symbols at the top of the page. The client chooses a symbol that goes with the given item as each question is read. One symbol will be left over and not used as an answer.

Objective: The client will choose an object associated with a given object.

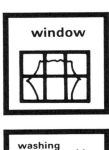

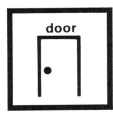

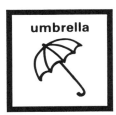

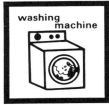

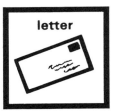

What goes with _____?

key

clothes

rain

rug

mailbox

131

Object Association

Directions: First review the symbols at the top of the page. The client chooses a symbol that goes with the given item as each question is read. One symbol will be left over and not used as an answer.

Objective: The client will choose an object associated with a given object.

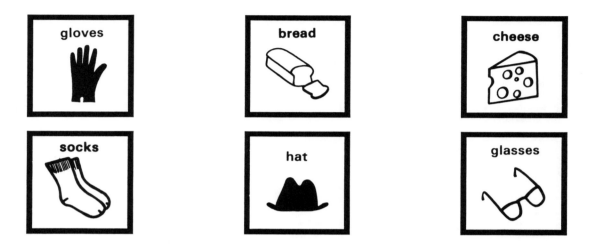

What goes with _____?

feet

head

toaster

eyes

hands

Object Association

Directions: First review the symbols at the top of the page. The client chooses a symbol that goes with the given item as each question is read. One symbol will be left over and not used as an answer.

Objective: The client will choose an object associated with a given object.

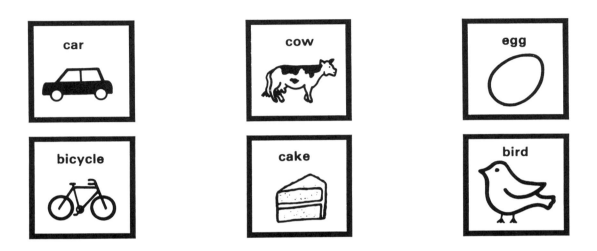

What goes with _____?

milk

gas

birthday

hen

worm

Object Association

Directions: First review the symbols at the top of the page. The client chooses a symbol that goes with the given item as each question is read. One symbol will be left over and not used as an answer.

Objective: The client will choose an object associated with a given object.

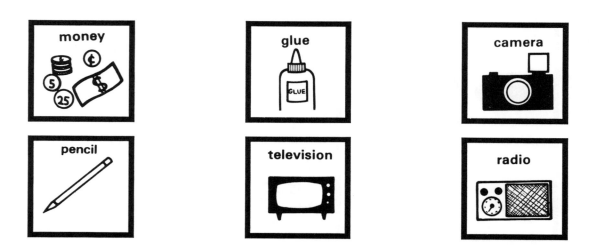

What goes with _____?

cartoons

bank

music

eraser

photo

Object Association

Directions: First review the symbols at the top of the page. The client chooses a symbol that goes with the given item as each question is read. One symbol will be left over and not used as an answer.

Objective: The client will choose an object associated with a given object.

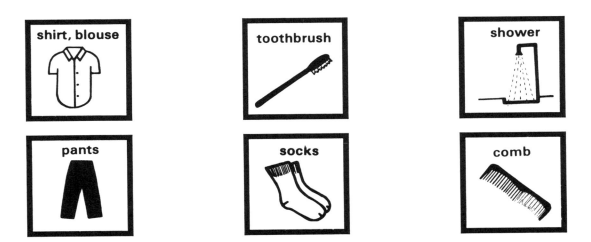

What goes with _____?

belt

brush

tie

shoes

toothpaste

135

Object Association

Directions: First review the symbols at the top of the page. The client chooses a symbol that goes with the given item as each question is read. One symbol will be left over and not used as an answer.

Objective: The client will choose an object associated with a given object.

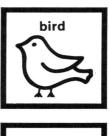

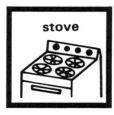

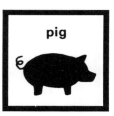

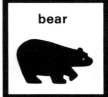

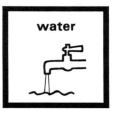

What goes with _____?

nest

farm

bowl

zoo

soap

136

Object Association

Directions: First review the symbols at the top of the page. The client chooses a symbol that goes with the given item as each question is read. One symbol will be left over and not used as an answer.

Objective: The client will choose an object associated with a given object.

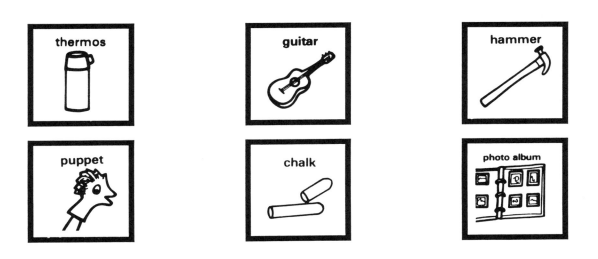

What goes with _____?

chalkboard

photos

lunch box

nails

music

Object Association

Directions: First review the symbols at the top of the page. The client chooses a symbol that goes with the given item as each question is read. One symbol will be left over and not used as an answer.

Objective: The client will choose an object associated with a given object.

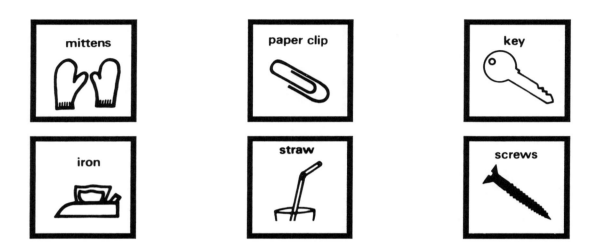

What goes with _____?

hands

lock

cup

ironing board

screwdriver

Object-Person Association

Directions: First review the symbols at the top of the page. The client chooses a person symbol who goes with the given item as each question is read.

Objective: The client will choose a person associated with a given object.

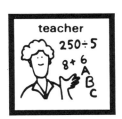

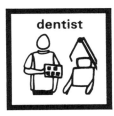

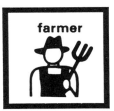

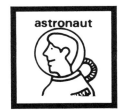

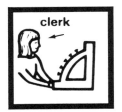

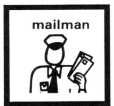

Who goes with _____?

barn

classroom

rocket

teeth

letters

store

139

Object-Person Association

Directions: First review the symbols at the top of the page. The client chooses a person symbol who goes with the given item as each question is read.

Objective: The client will choose a person associated with a given object.

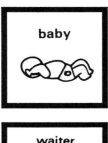

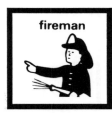

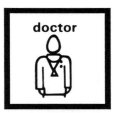

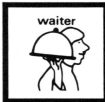

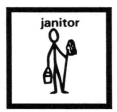

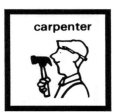

Who goes with _____?

medicine

restaurant

crib

fire engine

wood

vacuum cleaner

140

Part/Whole Association

Directions: First review the symbols at the top of the page. The client chooses a symbol to fill in the blank as each sentence is read. Some sentences may have more than one correct answer.

Objective: The client will choose all of the objects that contain a given part.

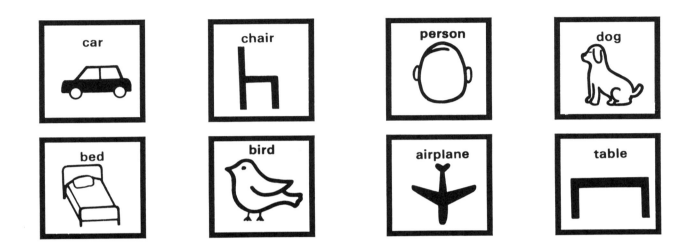

A leg is part of a _____.

A wheel is part of a _____.

Sheets are part of a _____.

Arms are part of a _____.

Hair is part of a _____.

A tail is part of a _____.

Part/Whole Association

Directions: First review the symbols at the top of the page. The client chooses a symbol to fill in the blank as each sentence is read. Some sentences may have more than one correct answer.

Objective: The client will choose all of the objects that contain a given part.

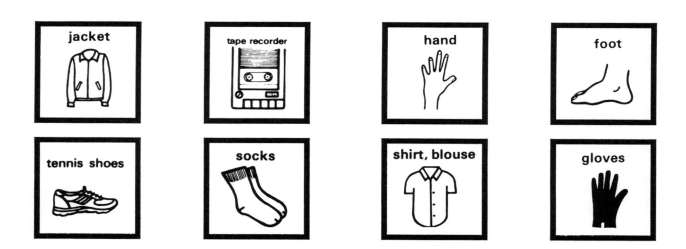

Laces are part of _____.

Sleeves are part of _____.

Fingers are part of _____.

Nails are part of _____.

Buttons are part of _____.

Toes are part of _____.

Part/Whole Association

Directions: First review the symbols at the top of the page. The client chooses a symbol to fill in the blank as each sentence is read. Some sentences may have more than one correct answer.

Objective: The client will choose all of the objects that contain a given part.

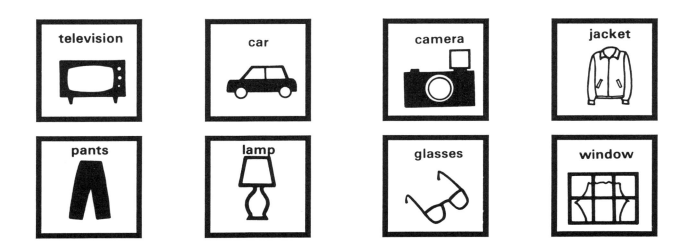

A hood is part of _____.

A screen is part of _____.

A trunk is part of _____.

A lens is part of _____.

A zipper is part of _____.

A light is part of _____.

Part/Whole Association

Directions: First review the symbols at the top of the page. The client chooses a symbol to fill in the blank as each sentence is read. Some sentences may have more than one correct answer.

Objective: The client will choose all of the objects that contain a given part.

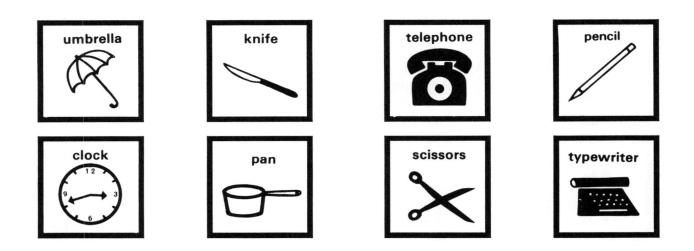

Numbers are part of _____.

Keys are part of _____.

An eraser is part of _____.

A point is part of _____.

A cord is part of _____.

A handle is part of _____.

144

Part/Whole Association

Directions: First review the symbols at the top of the page. The client chooses a symbol to fill in the blank as each sentence is read. Some sentences may have more than one correct answer.

Objective: The client will choose all of the objects that contain a given part.

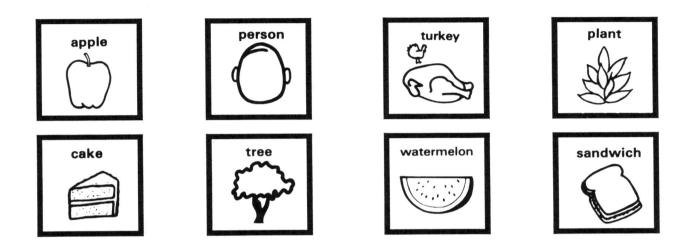

Bread is part of _____.

Frosting is part of _____.

A drumstick is part of _____.

Leaves are part of _____.

Seeds are part of _____.

Skin is part of _____.

145

Part/Whole Association

Directions: First review the symbols at the top of the page. The client chooses a symbol to fill in the blank as each sentence is read. Some sentences may have more than one correct answer.

Objective: The client will choose all of the objects that contain a given part.

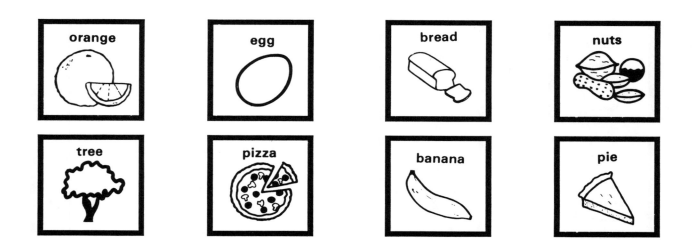

Crust is part of _____.

Cheese is part of _____.

A branch is part of _____.

A shell is part of _____.

A peel is part of _____.

A yolk is part of _____.

146

Part/Whole Association

Directions: First review the symbols at the top of the page. The client chooses a symbol to fill in the blank as each sentence is read. Some sentences may have more than one correct answer.

Objective: The client will choose all of the objects that contain a given part.

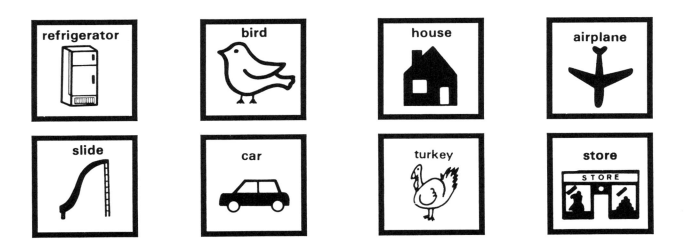

A door is part of _____.

A window is part of _____.

Feathers are part of _____.

A beak is part of _____.

Wings are part of _____.

Steps are part of _____.

147

Part/Whole Association

Directions: First review the symbols at the top of the page. The client chooses a symbol to fill in the blank as each sentence is read. Some sentences may have more than one correct answer.

Objective: The client will choose all of the objects that contain a given part.

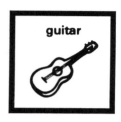
guitar

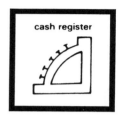
cash register

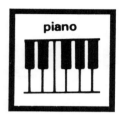
piano

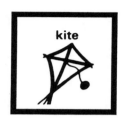
kite

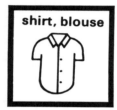
shirt, blouse

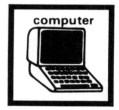
computer

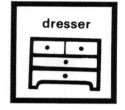
dresser

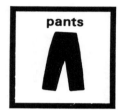
pants

A pocket is part of _____.

String is part of _____.

A drawer is part of _____.

Keys are part of _____.

A collar is part of _____.

Buttons are part of _____.

Location Analogies

Directions: First review the symbols at the top of the page. The client chooses a symbol to fill in the blank as each pair of sentences is read.

Objective: The client will choose a location to complete an analogy.

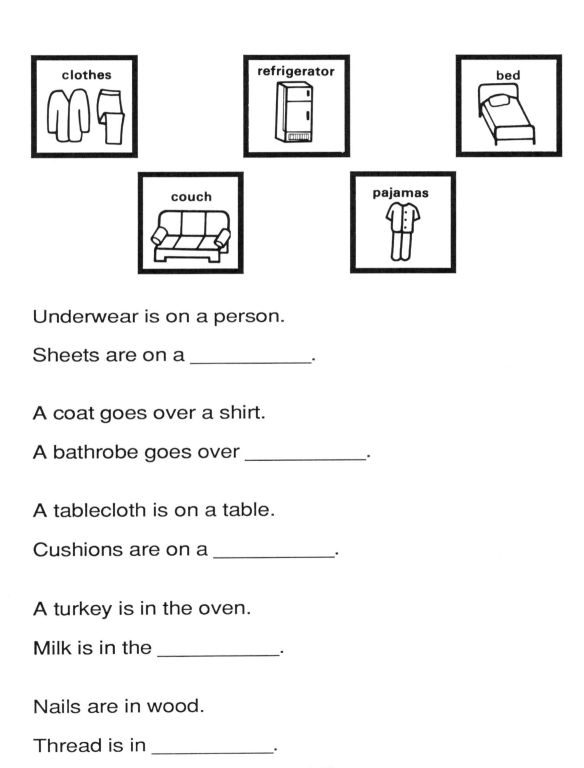

Underwear is on a person.

Sheets are on a _____.

A coat goes over a shirt.

A bathrobe goes over _____.

A tablecloth is on a table.

Cushions are on a _____.

A turkey is in the oven.

Milk is in the _____.

Nails are in wood.

Thread is in _____.

Location Analogies

Directions: First review the symbols at the top of the page. The client chooses a symbol to fill in the blank as each pair of sentences is read.

Objective: The client will choose a location to complete an analogy.

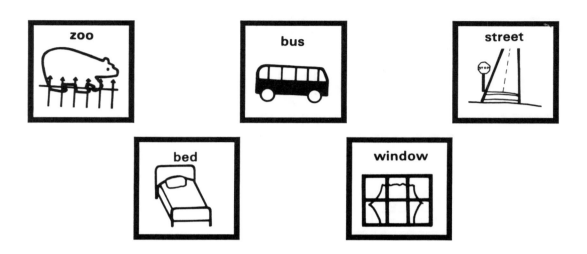

A train is on the track.

A car is on the _____.

A shade is on the lamp.

A curtain is on the _____.

Carpeting is on the floor.

A blanket is on the _____.

Chairs are in the house.

Seats are in a _____.

A cow lives on a farm.

A monkey lives in a _____.

Location Analogies

Directions: First review the symbols at the top of the page. The client chooses a symbol to fill in the blank as each pair of sentences is read.

Objective: The client will choose a location to complete an analogy.

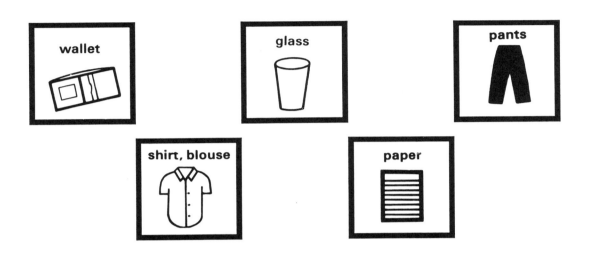

Belt loops are on pants.

A collar is on a _____.

Toothpaste is on a toothbrush.

Glue is on _____.

Flowers are in a vase.

A straw is in a _____.

A tie is on a shirt.

A belt is on _____.

Photographs are in an album.

Money is in a _____.

151

Location Analogies

Directions: First review the symbols at the top of the page. The client chooses a symbol to fill in the blank as each pair of sentences is read.

Objective: The client will choose a location to complete an analogy.

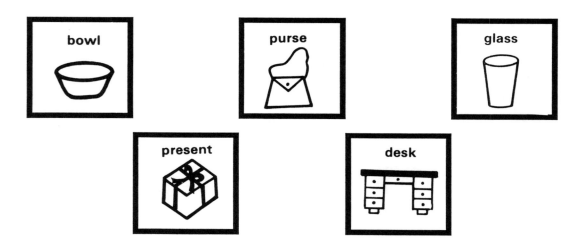

Soup is in a bowl.

Juice is in a _____.

A letter is in an envelope.

Files are in a _____.

Cards are in a deck.

A wallet is in a _____.

Coffee is in a cup.

Cereal is in a _____.

A stamp is on an envelope.

A bow is on a _____.

Location Analogies

Directions: First review the symbols at the top of the page. The client chooses a symbol to fill in the blank as each pair of sentences is read.

Objective: The client will choose a location to complete an analogy.

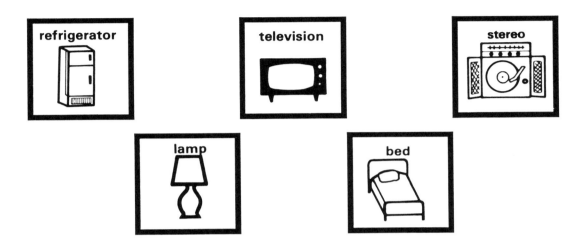

A cassette is in the tape recorder.

A record is on the _____.

Cushions are on the couch.

A pillow is on a _____.

Aspirin is in the medicine chest.

Cheese is in the _____.

An announcer is on the radio.

An actor is on _____.

Batteries are in a clock.

A lightbulb is in a _____.

Location Analogies

Directions: First review the symbols at the top of the page. The client chooses a symbol to fill in the blank as each pair of sentences is read.

Objective: The client will choose a location to complete an analogy.

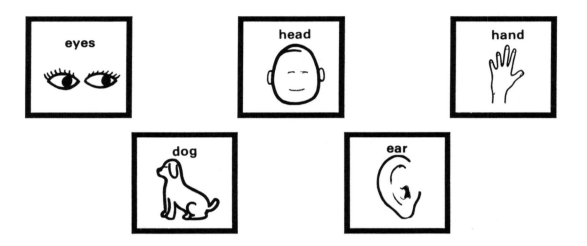

A necklace is on the neck.

An earring is on the _____.

Braces are on teeth.

Glasses are on _____.

Socks are on feet.

Gloves are on _____.

A bracelet is on a wrist.

A hat is on a _____.

A string is on a balloon.

A leash is on a _____.

Location Analogies

Directions: First review the symbols at the top of the page. The client chooses a symbol to fill in the blank as each pair of sentences is read.

Objective: The client will choose a location to complete an analogy.

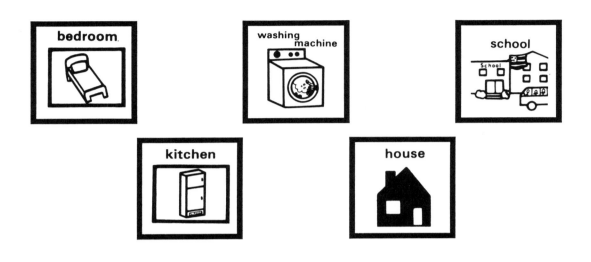

A bird lives in a nest.

A person lives in a _____.

A shower is in the bathroom.

A stove is in the _____.

Dirty dishes are in the sink.

Dirty clothes are in the _____.

The car is in the garage.

The bed is in the _____.

A doctor is in a hospital.

A teacher is in a _____.

Location Analogies

Directions: First review the symbols at the top of the page. The client chooses a symbol to fill in the blank as each pair of sentences is read.

Objective: The client will choose a location to complete an analogy.

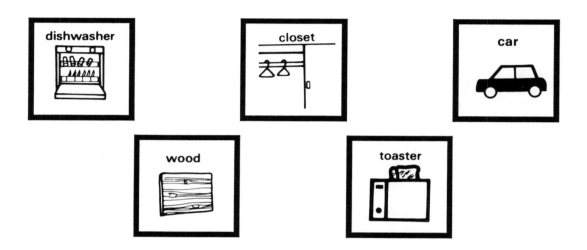

A book goes in the bookcase.

A jacket goes in the _____.

A belt is on pants.

A seatbelt is in a _____.

Clothing goes in the washing machine.

Silverware goes in the _____.

Staples go in paper.

Nails go in _____.

Soup is cooked in a pot.

Bread is cooked in a _____.

Action Analogies

Directions: First review the symbols at the top of the page. The client chooses a symbol to fill in the blank as each pair of sentences is read.

Objective: The client will choose an object to complete an action analogy.

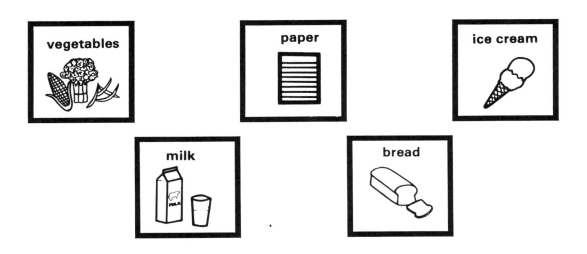

A shovel scoops sand.

A spoon scoops _____.

Sheep give wool.

Cows give _____.

Chalk writes on a blackboard.

A pencil writes on _____.

A nursery owner grows trees.

A farmer grows _____.

A butcher sells meat.

A baker sells_____.

157

Action Analogies

Directions: First review the symbols at the top of the page. The client chooses a symbol to fill in the blank as each pair of sentences is read.

Objective: The client will choose an object to complete an action analogy.

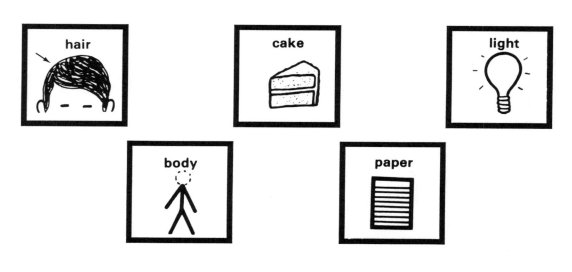

Detergent cleans clothes.

Soap cleans your _____.

A knob turns on the TV.

A switch turns on the _____.

A lawn mower cuts the grass.

A knife cuts _____.

A carpenter cuts wood.

A barber cuts _____.

A saw cuts wood.

Scissors cut _____.

Action Analogies

Directions: First review the symbols at the top of the page. The client chooses a symbol to fill in the blank as each pair of sentences is read.

Objective: The client will choose an object to complete an action analogy.

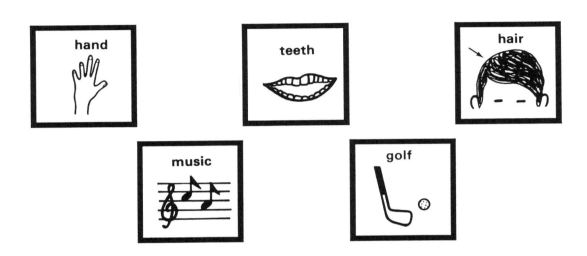

A hairbrush brushes hair.

A toothbrush brushes _____.

A TV plays movies.

A radio plays _____.

A dryer dries clothes.

A towel dries _____.

A musician plays the violin.

A golfer plays _____.

Soap cleans hands.

Shampoo cleans _____.

Action Analogies

Directions: First review the symbols at the top of the page. The client chooses a symbol to fill in the blank as each pair of sentences is read.

Objective: The client will choose an object to complete an action analogy.

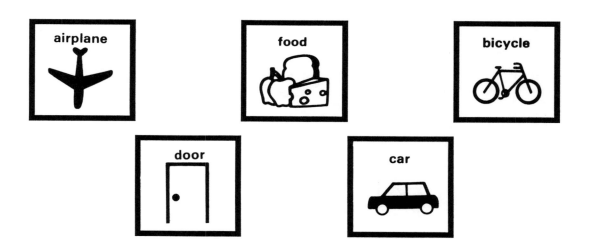

A key starts a car.

A pedal starts a _____.

A captain sails a boat.

A pilot flies a _____.

Handlebars turn a bike.

A steering wheel turns a _____.

A can opener opens cans.

A key opens a _____.

A carpenter builds with wood.

A cook cooks with _____.

160

Action Analogies

Directions: First review the symbols at the top of the page. The client chooses a symbol to fill in the blank as each pair of sentences is read.

Objective: The client will choose an object to complete an action analogy.

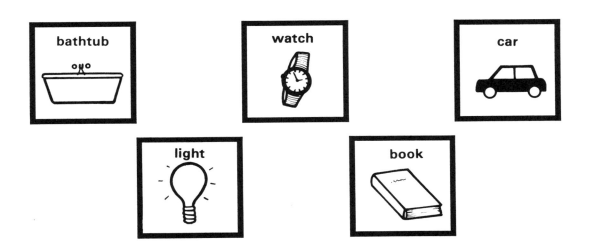

A repairman fixes the dryer.

A mechanic fixes the _____.

A roofer fixes the roof.

A jeweler fixes _____.

A repairman fixes washing machines.

An electrician fixes _____.

A poet writes poems.

An author writes a _____.

A repairman fixes TV's.

A plumber fixes _____.

Part/Whole Analogies

Directions: First review the symbols at the top of the page. The client chooses a symbol to fill in the blank as each pair of sentences is read.

Objective: The client will choose an object to complete a part/whole analogy.

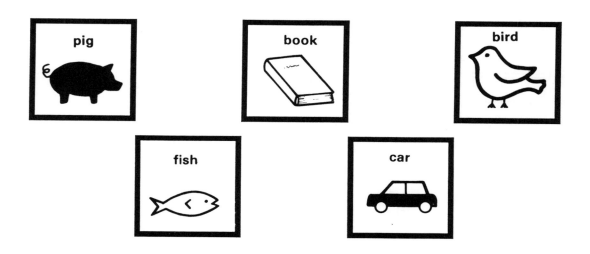

Songs are on a record.

Stories are in a _____.

A motor is in a boat.

An engine is in a _____.

Wings are on a bird.

Fins are on a _____.

A trunk is on an elephant.

A snout is on a _____.

Hair is on a person.

Feathers are on a _____.

Part/Whole Analogies

Directions: First review the symbols at the top of the page. The client chooses a symbol to fill in the blank as each pair of sentences is read.

Objective: The client will choose an object to complete a part/whole analogy.

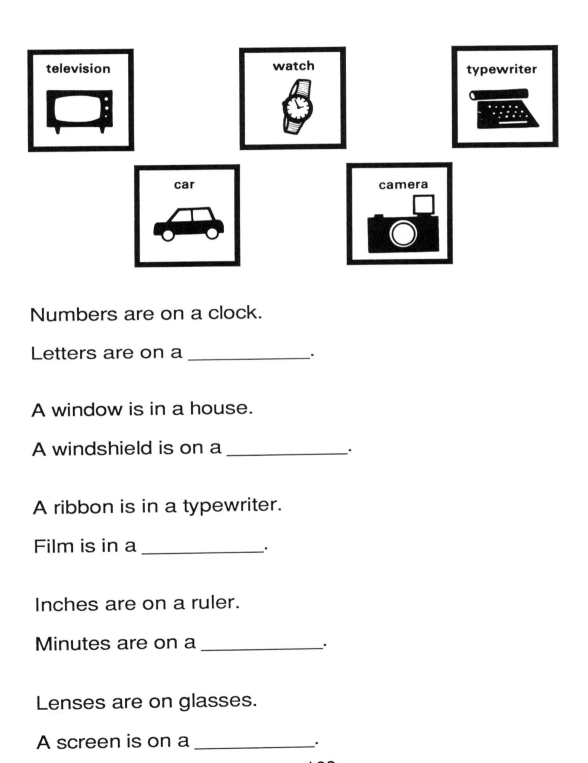

Numbers are on a clock.

Letters are on a _____.

A window is in a house.

A windshield is on a _____.

A ribbon is in a typewriter.

Film is in a _____.

Inches are on a ruler.

Minutes are on a _____.

Lenses are on glasses.

A screen is on a _____.

Part/Whole Analogies

Directions: First review the symbols at the top of the page. The client chooses a symbol to fill in the blank as each pair of sentences is read.

Objective: The client will choose an object to complete a part/whole analogy.

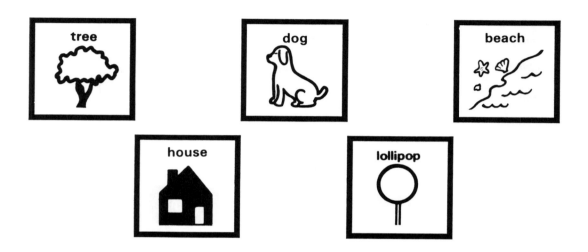

A string is on a kite.

A stick is on a _____.

Dirt is in the garden.

Sand is on the _____.

Petals are on a flower.

Leaves are on a _____.

The ceiling is in a room.

The roof is on a _____.

A stinger is on a bee.

A tail is on a _____.

Part/Whole Analogies

Directions: First review the symbols at the top of the page. The client chooses a symbol to fill in the blank as each pair of sentences is read.

Objective: The client will choose an object to complete a part/whole analogy.

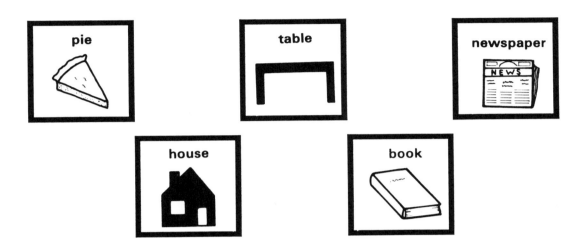

A frame is on a picture.

A cover is on a _____.

Chocolate chips are in cookies.

Fruit is in _____.

Chapters are in a book.

Articles are in a _____.

A trunk is in a car.

Closets are in a _____.

Wheels are on a car.

Legs are on a _____.

165

Part/Whole Analogies

Directions: First review the symbols at the top of the page. The client chooses a symbol to fill in the blank as each pair of sentences is read.

Objective: The client will choose an object to complete a part/whole analogy.

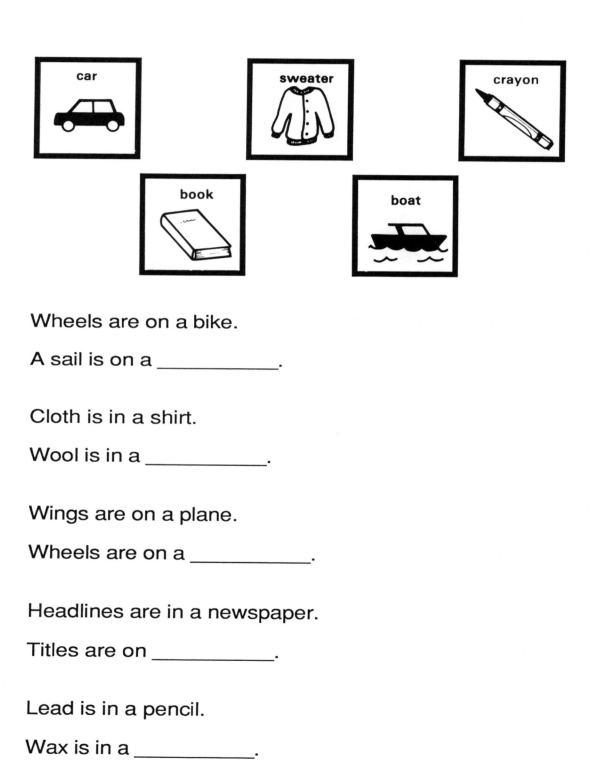

Wheels are on a bike.

A sail is on a _____.

Cloth is in a shirt.

Wool is in a _____.

Wings are on a plane.

Wheels are on a _____.

Headlines are in a newspaper.

Titles are on _____.

Lead is in a pencil.

Wax is in a _____.

Part/Whole Analogies

Directions: First review the symbols at the top of the page. The client chooses a symbol to fill in the blank as each pair of sentences is read.

Objective: The client will choose an object to complete a part/whole analogy.

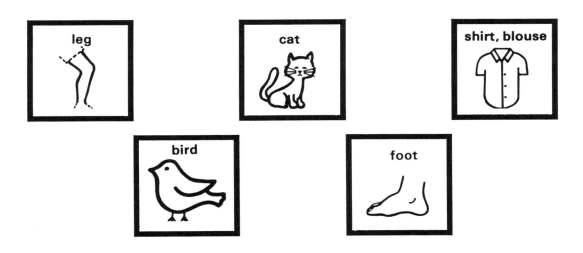

Fingers are on a hand.

Toes are on a _____.

Arms are on people.

Wings are on a _____.

Legs are on pants.

Sleeves are on a _____.

An elbow is on an arm.

A knee is on a _____.

Feet are on a person.

Paws are on a _____.

Part/Whole Analogies

Directions: First review the symbols at the top of the page. The client chooses a symbol to fill in the blank as each pair of sentences is read.

Objective: The client will choose an object to complete a part/whole analogy.

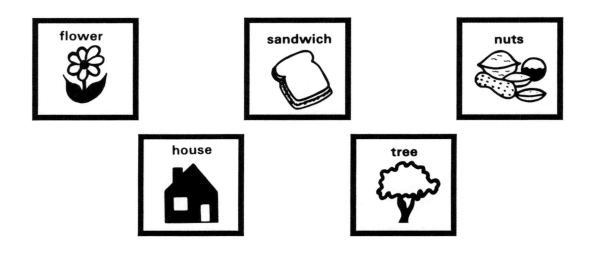

Flowers are on a plant.

Apples are on a _____.

Crust is on a pie.

Bread is on a _____.

A radio antenna is on a car.

A chimney is on a _____.

A peel is on an orange.

A shell is on a _____.

A trunk is on a tree.

A stem is on a _____.

Part/Whole Analogies

Directions: First review the symbols at the top of the page. The client chooses a symbol to fill in the blank as each pair of sentences is read.

Objective: The client will choose an object to complete a part/whole analogy.

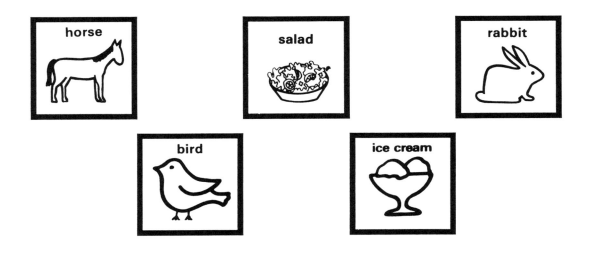

Hair is on a person.

Soft fur is on a _____.

A mouth is on a person.

A beak is on a _____.

Butter is on toast.

A cherry is on _____.

A shell is on a turtle.

A mane is on a _____.

Milk is in coffee.

Lettuce is in _____.

169

Part/Whole Analogies

Directions: First review the symbols at the top of the page. The client chooses a symbol to fill in the blank as each pair of sentences is read.

Objective: The client will choose an object to complete a part/whole analogy.

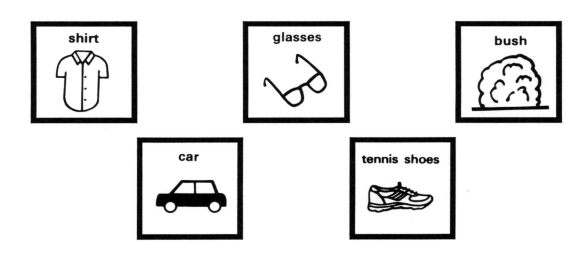

A zipper is on pants.

Buttons are on a _____.

Grapes are on a vine.

Berries are on a _____.

Strings are on a hood.

Laces are on _____.

A crystal is on a watch.

Lenses are on _____.

Handlebars are on a bike,

A steering wheel is on a _____.

Part/Whole Analogies

Directions: First review the symbols at the top of the page. The client chooses a symbol to fill in the blank as each pair of sentences is read.

Objective: The client will choose an object to complete a part/whole analogy.

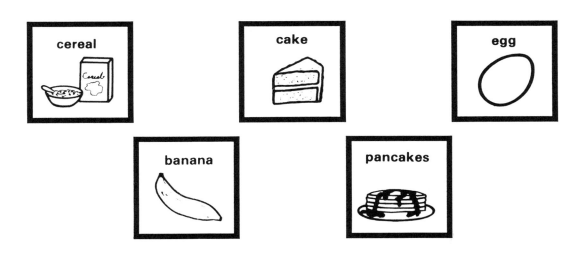

Dressing is on salad.

Syrup is on _____.

Skin is on an apple.

A peel is on a _____.

Sauce is on spaghetti.

Milk is in _____.

A core is in an apple.

A yolk is in an _____.

Cheese is on pizza.

Frosting is on a _____.

Part/Whole Analogies

Directions: First review the symbols at the top of the page. The client chooses a symbol to fill in the blank as each pair of sentences is read.

Objective: The client will choose an object to complete a part/whole analogy.

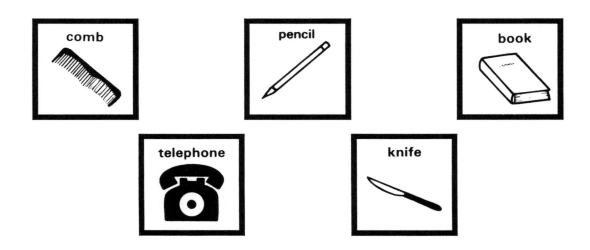

Pieces are in a puzzle.

Pages are in a _____.

Letters are on a typewriter.

Numbers are on a _____.

Prongs are on a fork.

An eraser is on a _____.

Bristles are on a brush.

Teeth are on a _____.

A point is on a pencil.

A blade is on a _____.

Whole/Part Analogies

Directions: First review the symbols at the top of the page. The client chooses a symbol to fill in the blank as each pair of sentences is read. One symbol will be left over and not used as an answer.

Objective: The client will choose an object to complete a whole/part analogy.

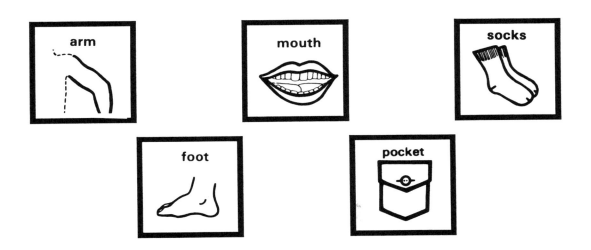

A bird has a beak.

A person has a _____.

Cats have paws.

People have _____.

A kangaroo has a pouch.

Pants have _____.

Birds have wings.

People have _____.

Whole/Part Analogies

Directions: First review the symbols at the top of the page. The client chooses a symbol to fill in the blank as each pair of sentences is read. One symbol will be left over and not used for an answer.

Objective: The client will choose an object to complete a whole/part analogy.

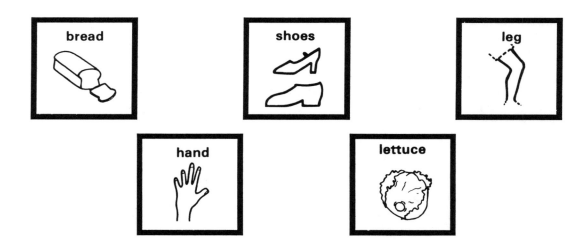

A leg has a foot.

An arm has a _____.

An egg has a shell.

A sandwich has _____.

A car has wheels.

A chair has _____.

Macaroni and cheese have noodles.

Salad has _____.

Whole/Part Analogies

Directions: First review the symbols at the top of the page. The client chooses a symbol to fill in the blank as each pair of sentences is read. One symbol will be left over and not used for an answer.

Objective: The client will choose an object to complete a whole/part analogy.

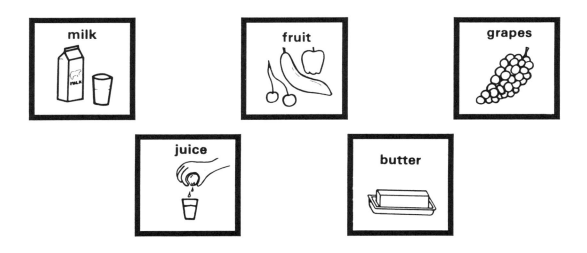

Spaghetti has sauce.

Cereal has _____.

A tree has apples.

A vine has _____.

Ice cream has syrup.

Toast has _____.

A stew has vegetables.

A pie has _____.

Component Analogies

Directions: First review the symbols at the top of the page. The client chooses a symbol to fill in the blank as each pair of sentences is read.

Objective: The client will choose a component item to complete an analogy.

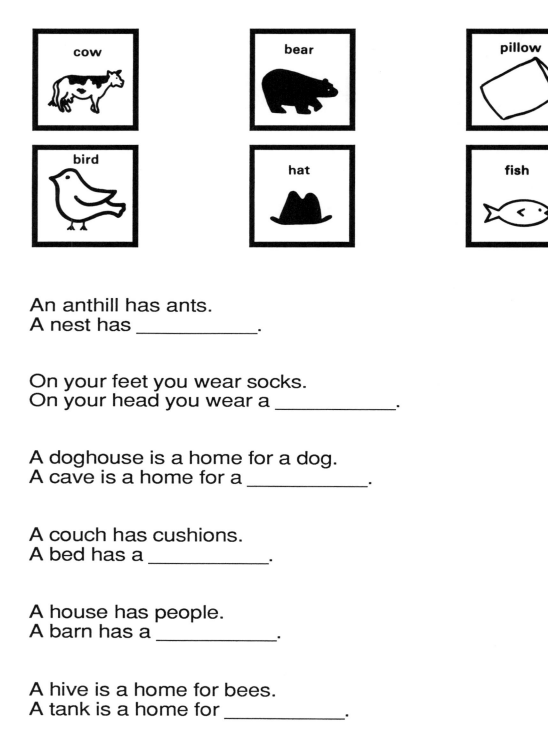

An anthill has ants.
A nest has _____.

On your feet you wear socks.
On your head you wear a _____.

A doghouse is a home for a dog.
A cave is a home for a _____.

A couch has cushions.
A bed has a _____.

A house has people.
A barn has a _____.

A hive is a home for bees.
A tank is a home for _____.

Component Analogies

Directions: First review the symbols at the top of the page. The client chooses a symbol to fill in the blank as each pair of sentences is read.

Objective: The client will choose a component item to complete an analogy.

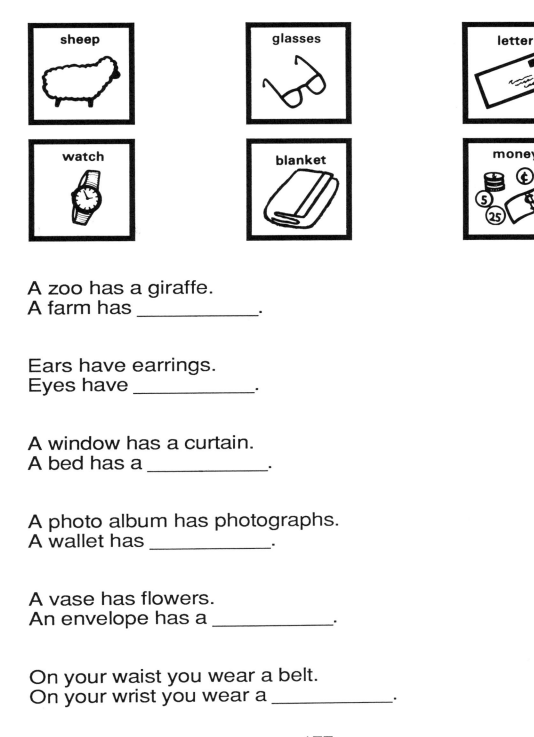

A zoo has a giraffe.
A farm has _____.

Ears have earrings.
Eyes have _____.

A window has a curtain.
A bed has a _____.

A photo album has photographs.
A wallet has _____.

A vase has flowers.
An envelope has a _____.

On your waist you wear a belt.
On your wrist you wear a _____.

Component Analogies

Directions: First review the symbols at the top of the page. The client chooses a symbol to fill in the blank as each pair of sentences is read.

Objective: The client will choose a component item to complete an analogy.

| ring | nail polish | water |
| table | drink | diaper |

Children have underwear.
Babies have _____.

A sandbox has sand.
A pool has _____.

On your wrist you wear a bracelet.
On your finger you wear a _____.

Lips have on lipstick.
Fingernails have on _____.

A hospital has beds.
A restaurant has _____.

A lunch bag has a sandwich.
A thermos has a _____.

178

If-then Completions

Directions: First review the symbols at the top of the page. The client chooses a symbol to fill in the blank as each sentence is read.

Objective: The client will choose a solution to complete an if-then statement.

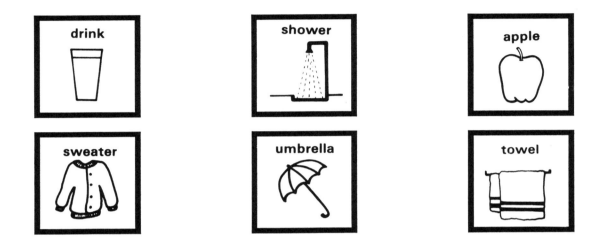

If it's raining, then take _____.

If you're hungry, then take _____.

If you're dirty, then take _____.

If you're wet, then take _____.

If you're cold, then take _____.

If you're thirsty, then take _____.

If-then Completions

Directions: First review the symbols at the top of the page. The client chooses a symbol to fill in the blank as each sentence is read.

Objective: The client will choose a solution to complete an if-then statement.

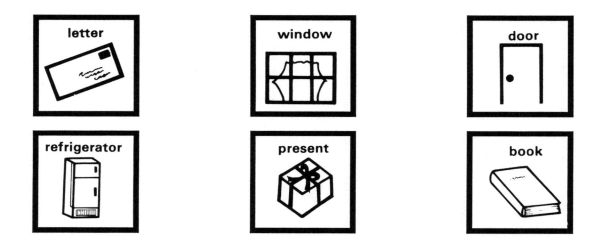

If you want milk, then open the _____.

If you're hot, then open the _____.

If it's your birthday, then open the _____.

If you want to read a story, then open the _____.

If you want to go outside, then open the _____.

If you want to read your mail, then open the _____.

If-then Completions

Directions: First review the symbols at the top of the page. The client chooses a symbol to fill in the blank as each sentence is read.

Objective: The client will choose a solution to complete an if-then statement.

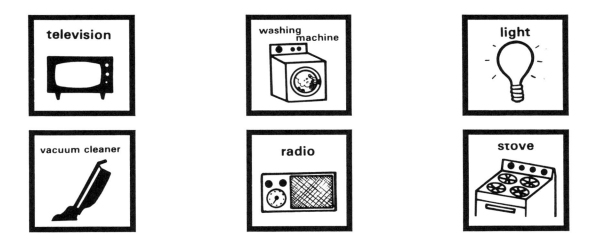

If it's dark, then turn on the _____.

If you want to watch a movie, then turn on the _____.

If you want to listen to music, then turn on the _____.

If you want to clean the floor, then turn on the _____.

If you want to cook eggs, then turn on the _____.

If you want to do laundry, then turn on the _____.

If-then Completions

Directions: First review the symbols at the top of the page. The client chooses a symbol to fill in the blank as each sentence is read.

Objective: The client will choose a solution to complete an if-then statement.

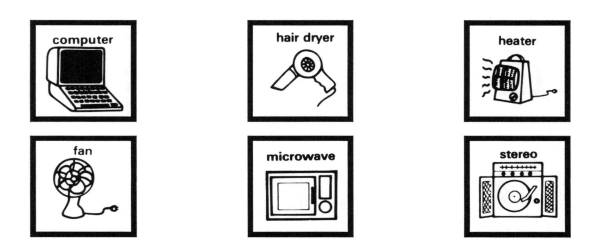

If you feel cold, then turn on the _____.

If you want to dry your wet hair, then turn on the _____.

If you want to cook food quickly, then turn on the _____.

If you want to play a record, then turn on the _____.

If you want to play a computer game, then turn on the _____.

If you feel too warm, then turn on the _____.

If-then Completions

Directions: First review the symbols at the top of the page. The client chooses a symbol to fill in the blank as each sentence is read.

Objective: The client will choose a solution to complete an if-then statement.

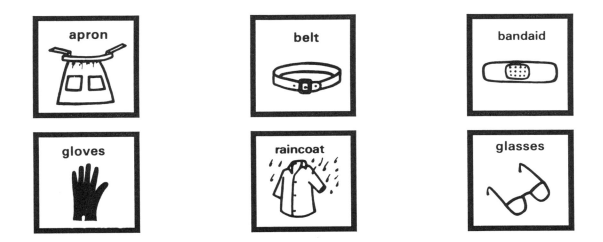

If you're going outside in the rain, then put on _____.

If you cut your finger, then put on _____.

If you don't want to get your clothes dirty when you cook, then put on _____.

If your pants are too loose, then put on _____.

If you want to keep your hands warm when it's cold, then put on _____.

If you want to see more clearly, then put on _____.

If-then Completions

Directions: First review the symbols at the top of the page. The client chooses a symbol to fill in the blank as each sentence is read.

Objective: The client will choose a solution to complete an if-then statement.

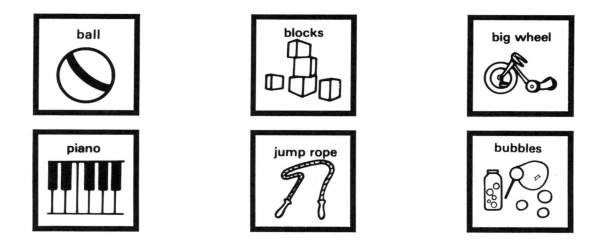

If you want to jump, then play with _____.

If you want to build a tower, then play with _____.

If you want to hear music, then play _____.

If you want to blow, then play with _____.

If you want to ride, then play with _____.

If you want to throw, then play with _____.

Determining Solutions

Directions: First review the symbols at the top of the page. The client chooses a symbol as each question is read. One symbol will be left over and not used as an answer.

Objective: The client will choose a solution to solve the stated problem.

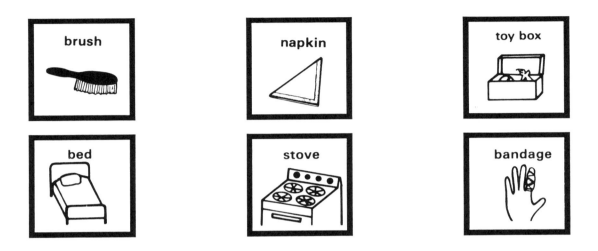

My mouth is dirty. What do I need?

I'm tired. What do I need?

My hair is a mess. What do I need?

My finger is bleeding. What do I need?

Clean up the toys. What do you need?

Determining Solutions

Directions: First review the symbols at the top of the page. The client chooses a symbol as each question is read. One symbol will be left over and not used as an answer.

Objective: The client will choose a solution to solve the stated problem.

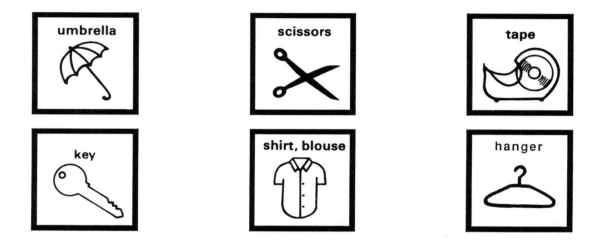

I ripped the paper. What do I need?

My coat is on the floor. What do I need?

The door is locked. What do I need?

The paper is too big. What do I need?

It's raining outside. What do I need?

Determining Solutions

Directions: First review the symbols at the top of the page. The client chooses a symbol as each question is read. One symbol will be left over and not used as an answer.

Objective: The client will choose a solution to solve the stated problem.

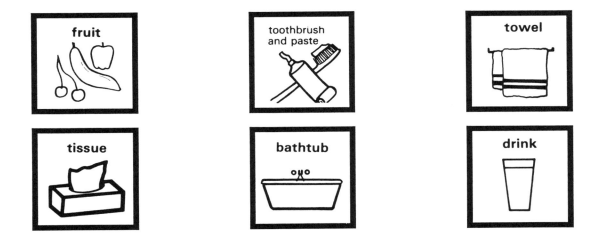

I'm thirsty. What do I need?

My nose is running. What do I need?

My teeth are dirty. What do I need?

My hands are wet. What do I need?

I'm hungry. What do I need?

Determining Solutions

Directions: First review the symbols at the top of the page. The client chooses a symbol as each question is read. One symbol will be left over and not used as an answer.

Objective: The client will choose a solution to solve the stated problem.

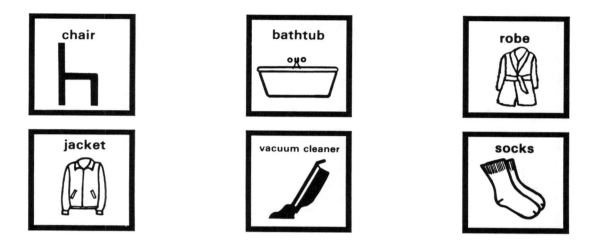

I can't stand up anymore. What do I need?

The carpet is dirty. What do I need?

It's cold out here. What do I need?

I'm all dirty. What do I need?

My feet are cold. What do I need?

Determining Solutions

Directions: First review the symbols at the top of the page. The client chooses a symbol as each question is read. One symbol will be left over and not used as an answer.

Objective: The client will choose a solution to solve the stated problem.

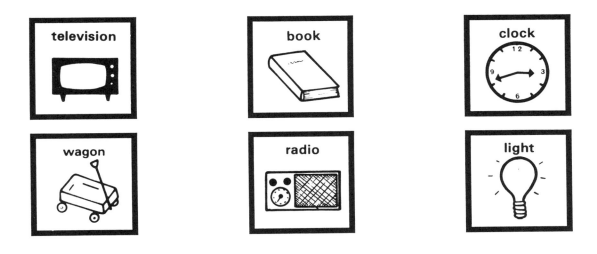

Give me a ride. What do you need?

It's too dark in here. What do I need?

Let's hear some music. What do we need?

I would like to know the time. What do I need?

Let's read a story. What do we need?

Determining Solutions

Directions: First review the symbols at the top of the page. The client chooses a symbol as each question is read. One symbol will be left over and not used as an answer.

Objective: The client will choose a solution to solve the stated problem.

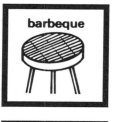

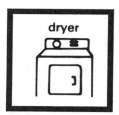

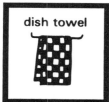

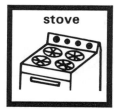

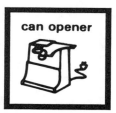

We want to cook hot dogs and hamburgers outside. What do we need?

I have to dry the dishes. What do I need?

I want to open a can of soup. What do I need?

I need to measure the milk for my recipe. What do I need?

My clothes are all wet from the rain. What do I need?

Determining Solutions

Directions: First review the symbols at the top of the page. The client chooses a symbol as each question is read. One symbol will be left over and not used as an answer.

Objective: The client will choose a solution to solve the stated problem.

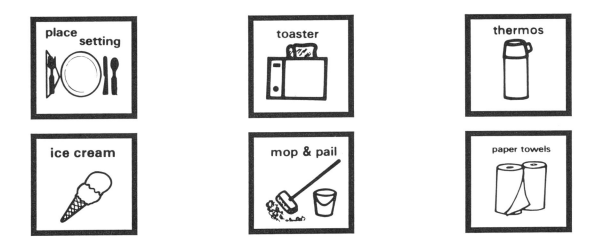

I want to toast my bread. What do I need?

I spilled juice on the table. What do I need?

I want to set the table. What do I need?

I want to take lemonade on the picnic. What do I need?

I want to wash the floor. What do I need?

Determining Solutions

Directions: First review the symbols at the top of the page. The client chooses a symbol as each question is read. One symbol will be left over and not used as an answer.

Objective: The client will choose a solution to solve the stated problem.

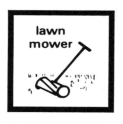

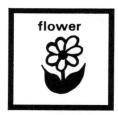

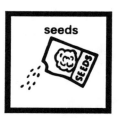

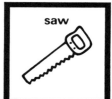

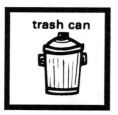

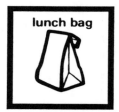

The grass is too high. What do I need?

I have to take out the garbage. What do I need?

I want to plant a vegetable garden. What do I need?

I want to cut this wood into pieces. What do I need?

I want to carry my sandwich and juice to school. What do I need?

Determining Solutions

Directions: First review the symbols at the top of the page. The client chooses a symbol as each question is read. One symbol will be left over and not used as an answer.

Objective: The client will choose a solution to solve the stated problem.

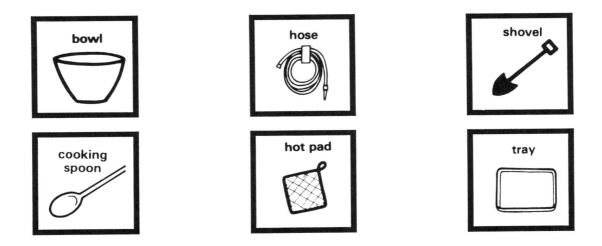

I have to stir the cake batter. What do I need?

I want to water the trees. What do I need?

I want to dig a hole. What do I need?

The waitress is carrying five plates of food to our table. What does she need?

I have to take the hot tray of cookies out of the oven. What do I need?

Determining Solutions

Directions: First review the symbols at the top of the page. The client chooses a symbol as each question is read. One symbol will be left over and not used as an answer.

Objective: The client will choose a solution to solve the stated problem.

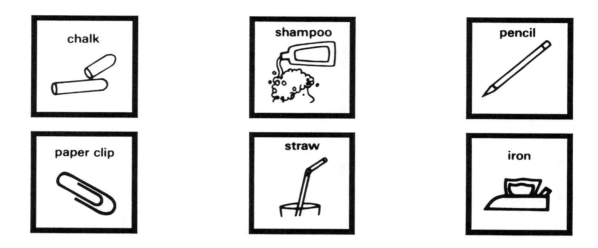

I want to wash my hair. What do I need?

The teacher wants to write on the blackboard. What does he need?

I want to drink my milkshake. What do I need?

I want to keep these papers together. What do I need?

My clothes are very wrinkled. What do I need?

Determining Solutions

Directions: First review the symbols at the top of the page. The client chooses a symbol as each question is read. One symbol will be left over and not used as an answer.

Objective: The client will choose a solution to solve the stated problem.

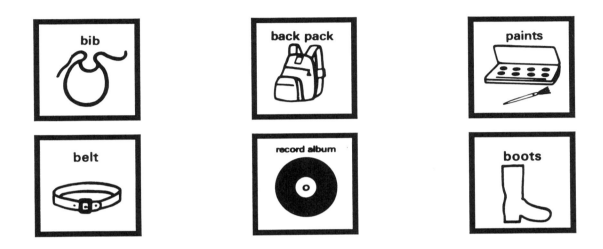

I want to play music on the stereo. What do I need?

I don't want the baby to get dirty when he eats. What do I need?

I have lots of books to carry to school. What do I need?

I want to make this drawing more colorful. What do I need?

I have to go outside in the snow. What do I need?

Choosing Items to Complete a Task

Directions: First review the symbols at the top of the page. Each question will have more than one correct answer. Encourage the client to find as many appropriate symbols as possible for each answer.

Objective: The client will choose the items necessary to complete a given task.

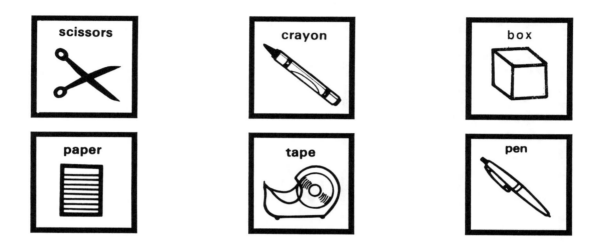

What do I need to write a letter?

What do I need to draw a picture?

What do I need to wrap a present?

Choosing Items to Complete a Task

Directions: First review the symbols at the top of the page. Each question will have more than one correct answer. Encourage the client to find as many appropriate symbols as possible for each answer.

Objective: The client will choose the items necessary to complete a given task.

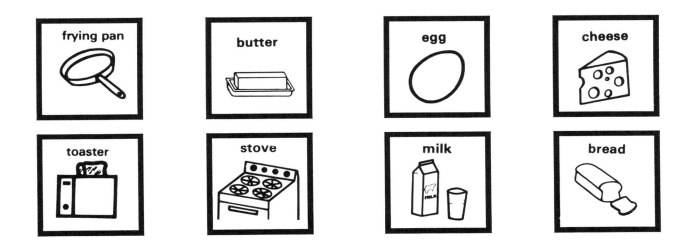

What do I need to make scrambled eggs?

What do I need to make toast?

What do I need to make a grilled cheese sandwich?

Choosing Items to Complete a Task

Directions: First review the symbols at the top of the page. Each question will have more than one correct answer. Encourage the client to find as many appropriate symbols as possible for each answer.

Objective: The client will choose the items necessary to complete a given task.

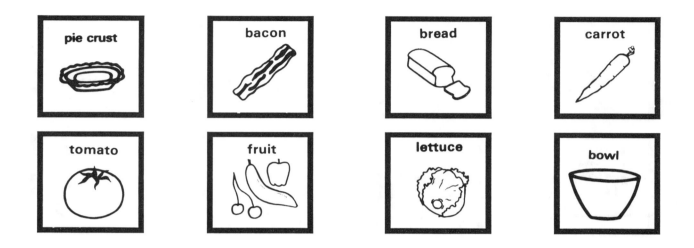

What do I need to make a fruit salad?

What do I need to make a bacon, lettuce, and tomato sandwich?

What do I need to make a pie?

What do I need to make a vegetable salad?

Choosing Items to Complete a Task

Directions: First review the symbols at the top of the page. Each question will have more than one correct answer. Encourage the client to find as many appropriate symbols as possible for each answer.

Objective: The client will choose the items necessary to complete a given task.

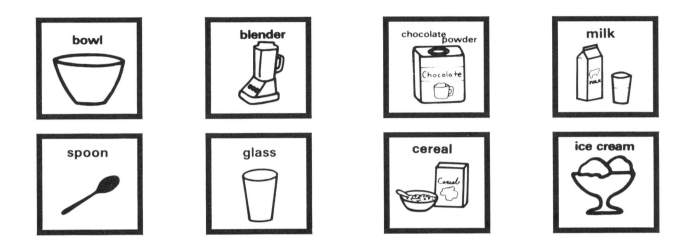

What do I need to make cold cereal?

What do I need to make chocolate milk?

What do I need to make a milkshake?

Choosing Items to Complete a Task

Directions: First review the symbols at the top of the page. Each question will have more than one correct answer. Encourage the client to find as many appropriate symbols as possible for each answer.

Objective: The client will choose the items necessary to complete a given task.

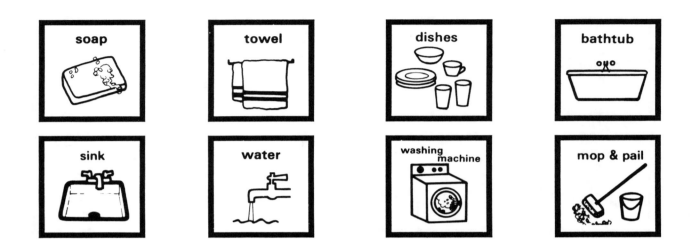

What do I need to take a bath?

What do I need to wash the dishes?

What do I need to do the laundry?

What do I need to wash the floor?

Choosing Items to Complete a Task

Directions: First review the symbols at the top of the page. Each question will have more than one correct answer. Encourage the client to find as many appropriate symbols as possible for each answer.

Objective: The client will choose the items necessary to complete a given task.

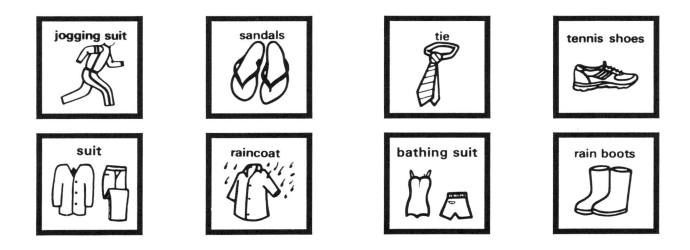

What should I wear to go to the beach?

What should John wear to go to a dinner party?

What should you wear to go outside in the rain?

What should I wear to go running in the park?

Determining Incorrect Information

Directions: First review the symbols at the top of the page. The client listens to the sentence as it is read. He/She then chooses a symbol that fits appropriately in the sentence to make it meaningful. If necessary, prompt the client by reading the sentence and pausing before the inappropriate word, encouraging the client to fill in the blank.

Objective: The client will choose an object to replace an incorrect object in the sentence.

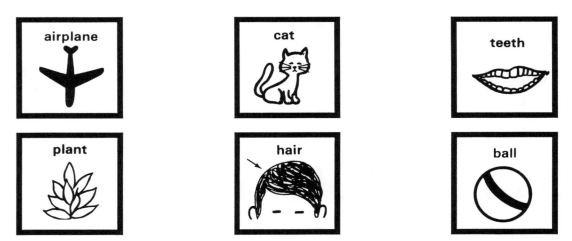

Water the lamp.

I brush my hair with a toothbrush.

Let's fly the car.

Throw the record to me.

"Meow," said the dog.

Determining Incorrect Information

Directions: First review the symbols at the top of the page. The client listens to the sentence as it is read. He/She then chooses a symbol that fits appropriately in the sentence to make it meaningful. If necessary, prompt the client by reading the sentence and pausing before the inappropriate word, encouraging the client to fill in the blank.

Objective: The client will choose an object to replace an incorrect object in the sentence.

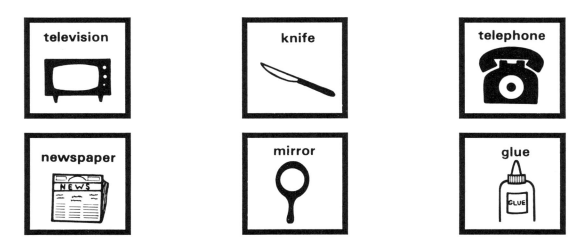

I like to read the TV.

I cut the cake with a scissors.

Take a look at yourself in the door.

Here's a hammer to fix the broken dish.

"Ring, ring." Answer the record player.

Determining Incorrect Information

Directions: First review the symbols at the top of the page. The client listens to the sentence as it is read. He/She then chooses a symbol that fits appropriately in the sentence to make it meaningful. If necessary, prompt the client by reading the sentence and pausing before the inappropriate word, encouraging the client to fill in the blank.

Objective: The client will choose an object to replace an incorrect object in the sentence.

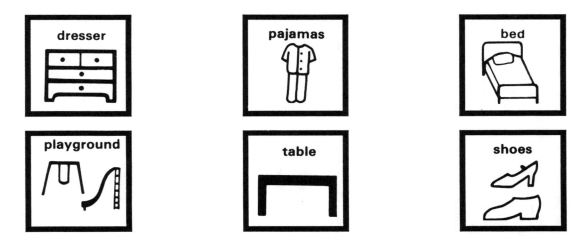

Put your gloves on your feet.

She goes to sleep on the table.

We went to the restaurant to play on the swings.

Put on your coat and go to bed.

Put your clothes away in the refrigerator.

Determining Incorrect Information

Directions: First review the symbols at the top of the page. The client listens to the sentence as it is read. He/She then chooses a symbol that fits appropriately in the sentence to make it meaningful. If necessary, prompt the client by reading the sentence and pausing before the inappropriate word, encouraging the client to fill in the blank.

Objective: The client will choose an object to replace an incorrect object in the sentence.

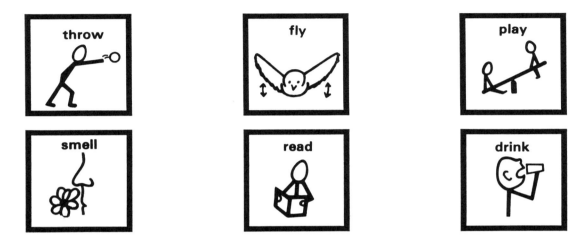

I like to listen to magazines.

We bought toys so the baby can work.

I eat juice.

Pull the ball.

These flowers taste good.

Determining Incorrect Information

Directions: First review the symbols at the top of the page. The client listens to the sentence as it is read. He/She then chooses a symbol that fits appropriately in the sentence to make it meaningful. If necessary, prompt the client by reading the sentence and pausing before the inappropriate word, encouraging the client to fill in the blank.

Objective: The client will choose an object to replace an incorrect object in the sentence.

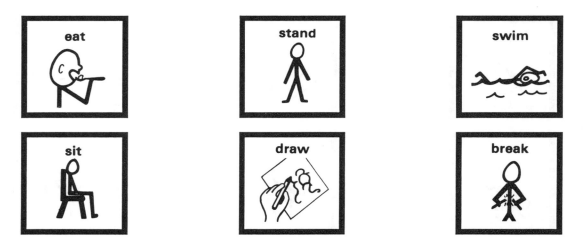

I dropped the plate and it started to cry.

Let's sleep at the restaurant.

Fish fly in the water.

We stand in the car.

It's fun to eat pictures.

Making Comparisons

Directions: First review the symbols at the top of the page. The client chooses a symbol from each of the two mentioned as the sentence is read.

Objective: The client will choose the object, from a group of two, that exhibits the stated attribute.

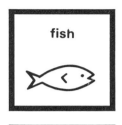
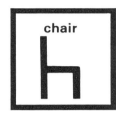
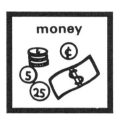

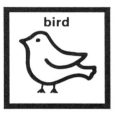

Which is louder, truck or typewriter?

Which is lighter, fish or truck?

Which is softer, chair or bird?

Which is quieter, bird or fish?

Which is heavier, money or truck?

Which is shinier, money or chair?

Making Comparisons

Directions: First review the symbols at the top of the page. The client chooses a symbol from each of the two mentioned as the sentence is read.

Objective: The client will choose the object, from a group of two, that exhibits the stated attribute.

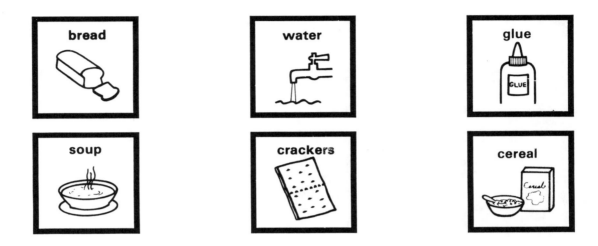

Which is thicker, water or glue?

Which is drier, cracker or soup?

Which is crunchier, bread or cracker?

Which is thinner, bread or cracker?

Which is stickier, glue or water?

Which is hotter, soup or cereal?

Making Comparisons

Directions: First review the symbols at the top of the page. The client chooses a symbol from each of the two mentioned as the sentence is read.

Objective: The client will choose the object, from a group of two, that exhibits the stated attribute.

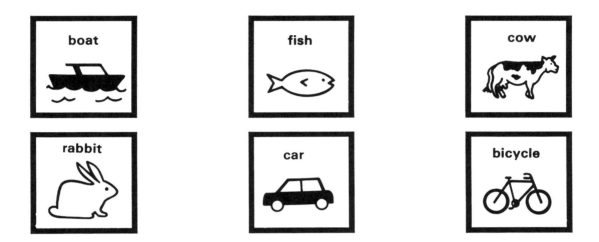

Which is faster, a car or a bike?

Which is smaller, a bike or a boat?

Which is softer, a rabbit or a car?

Which is slower, a cow or a rabbit?

Which is bigger, a cow or a rabbit?

Which is wetter, a fish or a boat?

Making Comparisons

Directions: First review the symbols at the top of the page. The client chooses a symbol from each of the two mentioned as the sentence is read.

Objective: The client will choose the object, from a group of two, that exhibits the stated attribute.

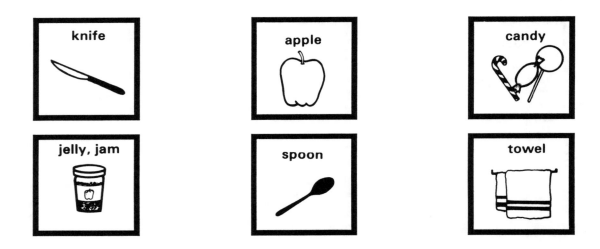

Which is shinier, a towel or a knife?

Which is sharper, a knife or a spoon?

Which is softer, a towel or an apple?

Which is harder, candy or jelly?

Which is stickier, jelly or an apple?

Which is more round, an apple or a spoon?

Making Comparisons

Directions: First review the symbols at the top of the page. The client chooses a symbol from each of the two mentioned as the sentence is read.

Objective: The client will choose the object, from a group of two, that exhibits the stated attribute.

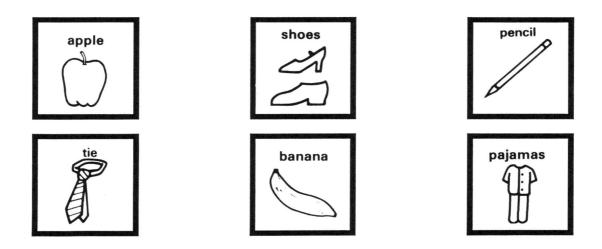

Which is softer, an apple or a banana?

Which is more round, an apple or a banana?

Which is sharper, a pencil or a tie?

Which is bigger, a tie or pajamas?

Which is smaller, shoes or pajamas?

Which is harder, pajamas or a pencil?

Making Comparisons

Directions: First review the symbols at the top of the page. The client chooses a symbol from each of the two mentioned as the sentence is read.

Objective: The client will choose the object, from a group of two, that exhibits the stated attribute.

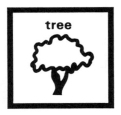
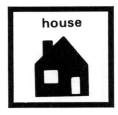
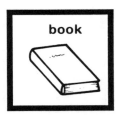
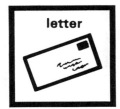
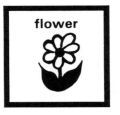
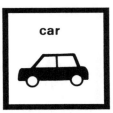

Which is thicker, a letter or a book?

Which is taller, a tree or a flower?

Which is lighter, a car or a letter?

Which is heavier, a tree or a book?

Which is thinner, a flower or a book?

Which is shorter, a car or a house?

Predicting an Outcome

Directions: First review the symbols at the top of the page. The client chooses a symbol to determine what will happen next after each group of sentences is read.

Objective: The client will choose the action that will occur following the situation described.

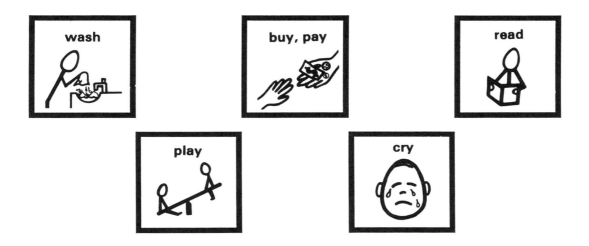

The baby finds a new toy. What will she do next?

You try on a great pair of shoes and they fit you just right. You want to get them. What will you do next?

Father finishes eating breakfast. He opens up the newspaper. What will he do next?

You look for some clean clothes to wear, but everything is dirty. What will you do next?

The baby falls down and bumps her head. What will she do next?

Predicting an Outcome

Directions: First review the symbols at the top of the page. The client chooses a symbol to determine what will happen next after each group of sentences is read.

Objective: The client will choose the action that will occur following the situation described.

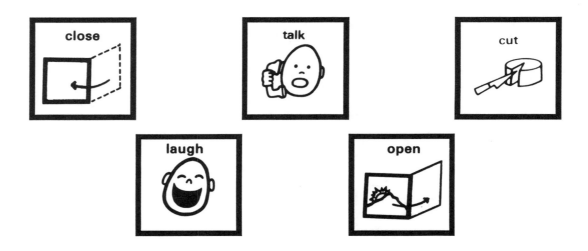

You call up a friend on the phone. He answers. What will you do next?

You pick up all the papers that were blown around by the wind. You notice that the window is open. What will you do next?

Brian blows out the candles on his birthday cake. Everyone wants a piece. What will he do next?

You listen to someone tell a very funny joke. What will you do next?

George wants to make some soup. He takes a can of soup. What will he do next?

Predicting an Outcome

Directions: First review the symbols at the top of the page. The client chooses a symbol to determine what will happen next after each group of sentences is read.

Objective: The client will choose the action that will occur following the situation described.

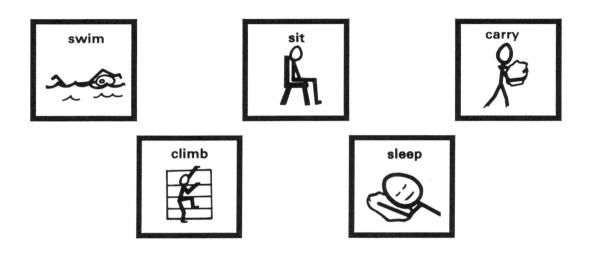

You're out walking with your small dog. He hurts his paw and can't walk. What will you do next?

Father needs to fix the roof. He leans the ladder up against the house. What will he do next?

You're tired of standing. What will you do next?

Katie is sitting beside a swimming pool. She's hot and wants to cool off. What will she do next?

You're tired and it's late at night. What will you do next?

Predicting an Outcome

Directions: First review the symbols at the top of the page. The client chooses a symbol to determine what will happen next after each group of sentences is read.

Objective: The client will choose the action that will occur following the situation described.

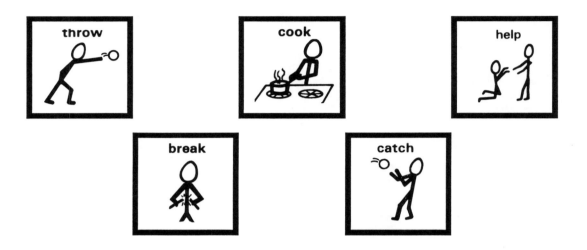

You have the ball. Brad is waiting to catch it. What will you do next?

Your friend is having trouble opening a jar. What will you do next?

Someone bumps into Kevin when he's carrying too many plates. What will happen next?

You see a ball coming towards you. What will you do next?

You've invited a lot of people for dinner. Dinner is not ready. What will you do next?

Predicting an Outcome

Directions: First review the symbols at the top of the page. The client chooses a symbol to determine what will happen next after each group of sentences is read.

Objective: The client will choose the action that will occur following the situation described.

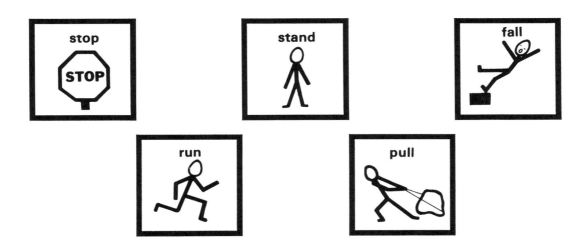

You put your books too close to the edge of the table. What will happen next?

Karen is playing the piano. Her father yells that he is trying to sleep. What will she do next?

You're playing with your wagon and Billy climbs in. He wants a ride. What will you do next?

You can't reach the book on the shelf because you're sitting down. What will you do next?

You are walking to the bus stop. You see that the bus is about to leave. What will you do next?

Predicting an Outcome

Directions: First review the symbols at the top of the page. The client chooses a symbol to determine what will happen next after each group of sentences is read.

Objective: The client will choose the action that will occur following the situation described.

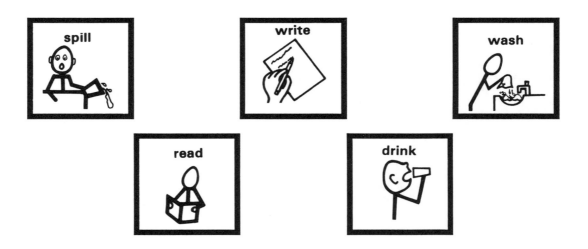

The spicy pizza sure makes Susan thirsty. What will she do next?

The cat bumps into the jar of paint and it begins to fall. What will happen next?

You bought a card to send to your friend. You need to put your name on the card. What will you do next?

You finish cleaning out the garage and your hands are very dirty. It's time for dinner. What will you do next?

Mary takes a book from the shelf. What will she do next?

Predicting an Outcome

Directions: First review the symbols at the top of the page. The client chooses a symbol to determine what will happen next after each group of sentences is read.

Objective: The client will choose the action that will occur following the situation described.

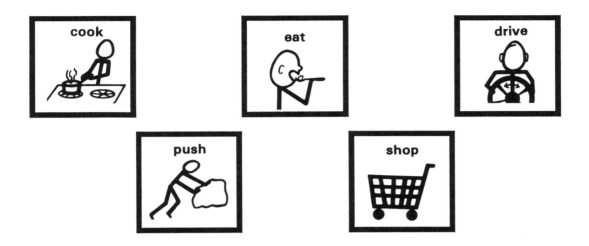

You need to buy food. You go to the store. What will you do next?

The mother puts her baby on the swing. The swing is not moving. What will she do next?

Brittany is hungry. She takes a frozen dinner out of the freezer. What will she do next?

The bus driver stops at the bus stop. The people waiting get on the bus. What will the bus driver do next?

Harry finishes working and is hungry. What will he do next?

Predicting an Outcome

Directions: First review the symbols at the top of the page. The client chooses a symbol to determine what will happen next after each group of sentences is read.

Objective: The client will choose the action that will occur following the situation described.

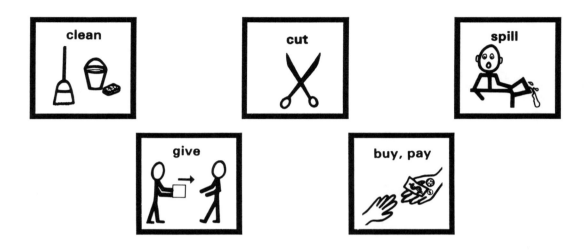

You have a present for Joe. Joe rings the doorbell and comes in. What will you do next?

Sarah wants a small piece of paper and all she can find is a large piece. What will she do next?

Margaret waters her plants and spills the water all over the floor. What will she do next?

You start to bake a cake. You need three eggs, but only have one. What will you do next?

Fred's elbow knocks against your glass of juice. What will happen next?

Predicting an Outcome

Directions: First review the symbols at the top of the page. The client chooses a symbol to determine what will happen next after each group of sentences is read.

Objective: The client will choose the action that will occur following the situation described.

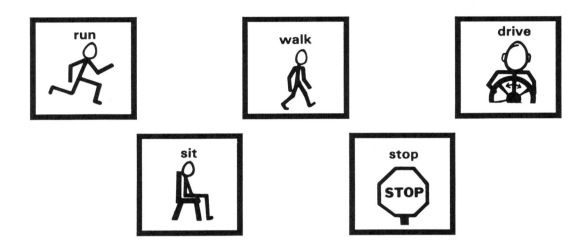

You have work to do. You walk over to your desk and pull out the chair. What will you do next?

Tom needs to go to the store. He gets in his car. What will Tom do next?

The runners are lined up at the starting line. The whistle is blown. What will they do next?

You decide to go to a friend's house. It's close by so you don't have to drive. What will you do next?

You're driving and the traffic light turns red. What will you do next?

Predicting an Outcome

Directions: First review the symbols at the top of the page. The client chooses a symbol to determine what will happen next after each group of sentences is read.

Objective: The client will choose the action that will occur following the situation described.

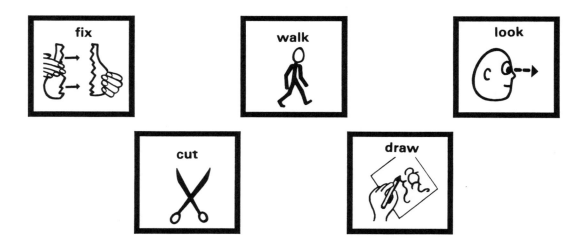

You've entered a poster contest. The best picture wins a prize. You have paper and magic markers. What will you do next?

Joe lost his watch. What will he do next?

Christine's school is very close to home, so she doesn't have to take a bus. After she eats her breakfast, it's time to go to school. What will she do next?

You drop your eyeglasses and they break. What will you do next?

Bob's picture is in the newspaper. He would like to save his picture, but not the whole page. What will he do next?

Predicting an Outcome

Directions: First review the symbols at the top of the page. The client chooses a symbol to determine what will happen next after each group of sentences is read.

Objective: The client will choose the action that will occur following the situation described.

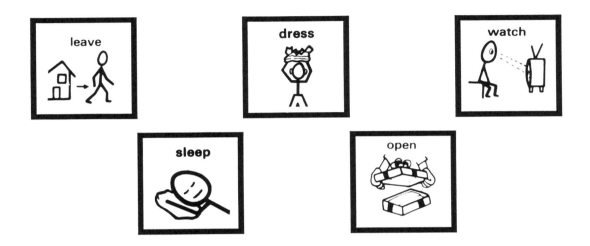

Sally gives you a birthday present. It's wrapped and has a bow on it. What will happen next?

Ken has ten minutes to get to school. He's still in his pajamas. What will he do next?

You turn on the TV. What will you do next?

It's time for the baby to take a nap. What will he do next?

You're finishing your drink. The restaurant is closing. What will you do next?

Predicting an Outcome

Directions: First review the symbols at the top of the page. The client chooses a symbol to determine what will happen next after each group of sentences is read.

Objective: The client will choose the action that will occur following the situation described.

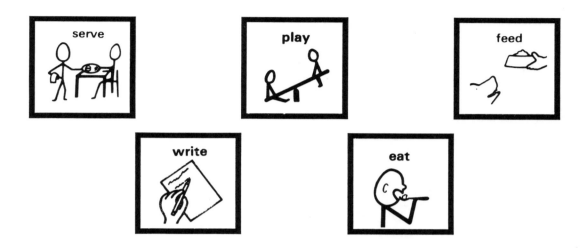

The members of the basketball team go out on the court. What will they do next?

You receive a letter from your friend Kathy. You want to answer her right away. What will you do next?

Jim's dog is hungry. Jim opens a can of dog food. What will he do next?

Rose orders a hamburger in the restaurant. A few minutes later, the waiter comes out of the kitchen carrying a tray. What will he do next?

You feel hungry during the movie. You buy a carton of popcorn and go back to your seat. What will you do next?

Predicting an Outcome

Directions: First review the symbols at the top of the page. The client chooses a symbol to determine what will happen next after each group of sentences is read.

Objective: The client will choose the action that will occur following the situation described.

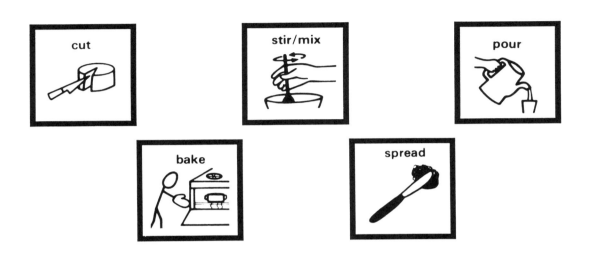

You take out bread and peanut butter to make a sandwich. You open the peanut butter jar and scoop some out with the knife. What will you do next?

You and your friends are thirsty. You get a pitcher of juice from the refrigerator and three empty glasses. What will you do next?

Kelly takes the last piece of cake, but her sister says she wants some too. Kelly wants to share the cake. What will she do next?

Jenny is making a cake. The recipe says to stir the ingredients until all the lumps are gone. Jenny looks in the bowl and sees lumps. What will she do next?

Mark puts the rest of the fruit into the pie crust. He opens the oven door. What will he do next?

Drawing Conclusions

Directions: First review the symbols at the top of the page. The client chooses one or more symbols to fill in the missing information from each paragraph. Some questions should be answered with two word phrases. One or two symbols may be left over and not used as answers.

Objective: After hearing a partial description of a situation, the client will determine the missing information to draw a conclusion.

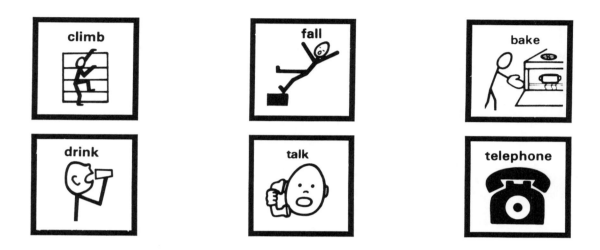

Sarah has no dessert to eat. She mixes eggs, butter, and flour in a bowl. After dinner, she eats a piece of cake. How can Sarah eat cake if there was no dessert?

Pam is climbing a tree. She goes higher and higher. Then Pam is sitting at the bottom of the tree. Her knee and her arm are hurt. Why do you think Pam is sitting on the ground with her knee and her arm hurt?

Mark is playing outside. He sees a house on fire. He runs inside his house. Next, fire engines are racing down the street to the fire. What do you think Mark did in his house?

Drawing Conclusions

Directions: First review the symbols at the top of the page. The client chooses one or more symbols to fill in the missing information from each paragraph. Some questions should be answered with two word phrases. One or two symbols may be left over and not used as answers.

Objective: After hearing a partial description of a situation, the client will determine the missing information to draw a conclusion.

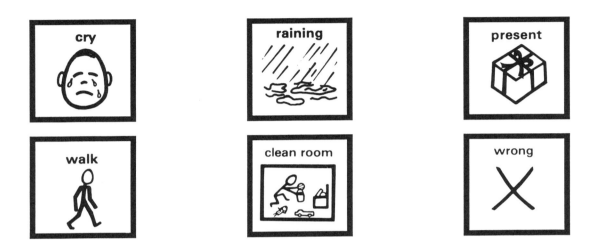

Dave goes outside for a walk. After a while he hears thunder. By the time Dave gets home, he is all wet. Why do you think Dave is all wet?

Mom says Justin can't go outside until his room is clean. He cries. Later Mom is smiling and lets Justin go outside. Why do you think Justin is going outside now?

Bobby goes to the bookstore and buys a book. He wraps it and takes the book to a friend's house. Why do you think Bobby brings the book to a friend's house?

Ruth is writing answers on her paper. Next she's erasing what she wrote. Why do you think she's erasing her answers?

Drawing Conclusions

Directions: First review the symbols at the top of the page. The client chooses one or more symbols to fill in the missing information from each paragraph. Some questions should be answered with two word phrases. One or two symbols may be left over and not used as answers.

Objective: After hearing a partial description of a situation, the client will determine the missing information to draw a conclusion.

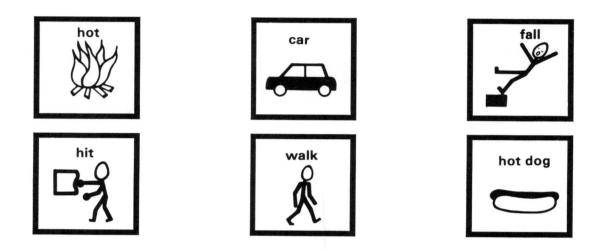

Bert is playing ball. His ball rolls into the street. Bert runs into the street and suddenly stops. Why do you think he stops?

Mom takes the cookies out of the oven. When she's not looking, Brian takes a cookie. "Ow!" he yells and drops the cookie. Why do you think Brian yells and drops the cookie?

Sam makes a big house out of blocks. Tony comes running through the room. Sam's blocks are scattered all over the floor. Why do you think the blocks are scattered all over the floor?

Pat puts her hot dog on a bun. She takes a bite, but doesn't taste the hot dog. Suddenly, her father slips and falls right beside her. Why do you think her father slips and falls?

Drawing Conclusions

Directions: First review the symbols at the top of the page. The client chooses one or more symbols to fill in the missing information from each paragraph. Some questions should be answered with two word phrases. One or two symbols may be left over and not used as answers.

Objective: After hearing a partial description of a situation, the client will determine the missing information to draw a conclusion.

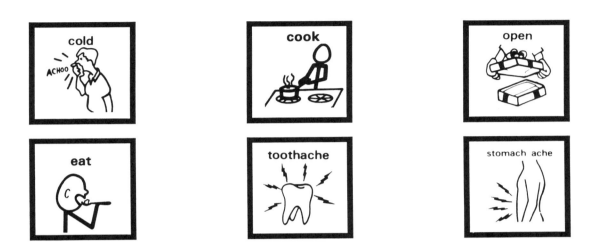

Pete keeps sneezing and coughing. He takes some cough medicine. Then he asks his mother to buy him more tissues. Why do you think he takes medicine and wants more tissues?

Melissa's mouth is swollen and it hurts when she tries to eat. She calls the dentist. Why do you think she calls the dentist?

Lisa shuts off the oven and takes out the casserole dish. Then she sets the table and calls her family into the room. Why do you think she calls her family together?

Barry looks around at the birthday presents his friends brought him. He tries to guess what is inside each box. Barry looks happy. He holds up a racing car that he's been wanting. How do you think he knows what one of his presents is?

Drawing Conclusions

Directions: First review the symbols at the top of the page. The client chooses one or more symbols to fill in the missing information from each paragraph. Some questions should be answered with two word phrases. One or two symbols may be left over and not used as answers.

Objective: After hearing a partial description of a situation, the client will determine the missing information to draw a conclusion.

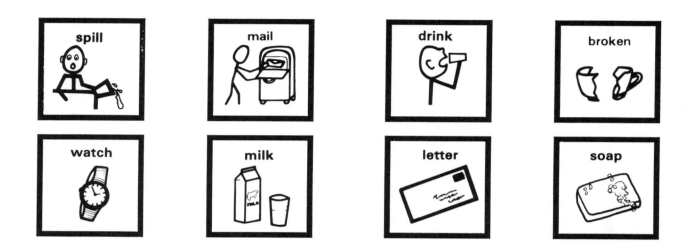

Barbara puts away her paper, pen, and envelopes. She looks out the window and waits for the mailman to come. Why do you think Barbara is waiting for the mailman?

Ben pours a glass of juice. He puts it next to a glass full of soapy bubbles. Ben takes a drink but quickly spits it out. Why do you think Ben spits out his drink?

Vanessa is drinking milk and eating cookies. She reaches across the table for another cookie. Mom looks angry. She starts mopping the floor. Why do you think Mom is mopping the floor?

Robin is going to the movies at 2:00 o'clock. She looks at her watch. It's 12:00 o'clock. She eats lunch and reads a story. Then she looks at her watch again. It's 12:00 o'clock. Why does Robin think the time on her watch hasn't changed?

Memory for Related Words

Directions: First review the symbols at the top of the page. The client touches the symbol after each word is read.

Objective: The client will repeat one word after it is presented.

Food

pretzel	soup	bread
cheese	carrot	hot dog

carrot; _____

pretzel; _____

bread; _____

cheese; _____

hot dog; _____

soup; _____

Memory for Related Words

Directions: First review the symbols at the top of the page. The client touches the symbol after each word is read.

Objective: The client will repeat one word after it is presented.

Clothes

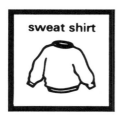

sweat shirt

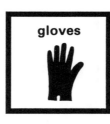

gloves

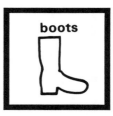

boots

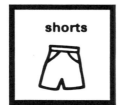

shorts

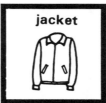

jacket

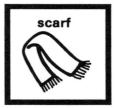

scarf

gloves; _____

shorts; _____

sweatshirt; _____

boots; _____

jacket; _____

scarf; _____

Memory for Related Words

Directions: First review the symbols at the top of the page. The client touches the symbol after each word is read.

Objective: The client will repeat one word after it is presented.

Furniture

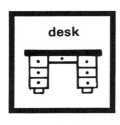

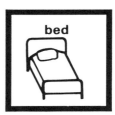

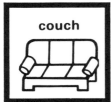

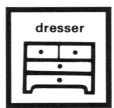

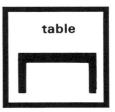

lamp; _____

couch; _____

table; _____

desk; _____

bed; _____

dresser; _____

Memory for Related Words

Directions: First review the symbols at the top of the page. The client touches the symbol after each word is read.

Objective: The client will repeat one word after it is presented.

Bedroom Items

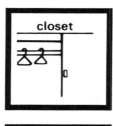

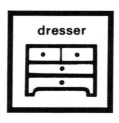

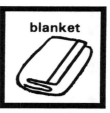

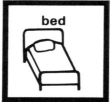

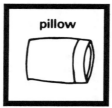

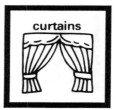

bed; _____

blanket; _____

dresser; _____

closet; _____

curtains; _____

pillow; _____

Memory for Related Words

Directions: First review the symbols at the top of the page. The client touches the symbol after each word is read.

Objective: The client will repeat one word after it is presented.

Playthings

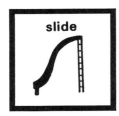
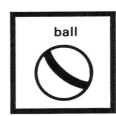
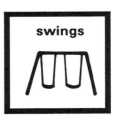
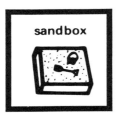
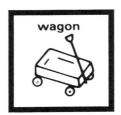
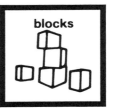

sand box; _____

wagon; _____

slide; _____

blocks; _____

ball; _____

swings; _____

Memory for Related Words

Directions: First review the symbols at the top of the page. The client touches the symbol after each word is read.

Objective: The client will repeat one word after it is presented.

Vegetables

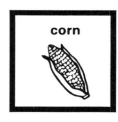

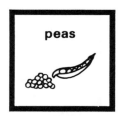

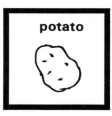

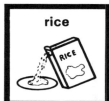

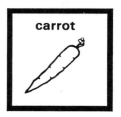

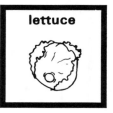

peas; _____

lettuce; _____

corn; _____

rice; _____

carrot; _____

potato; _____

Memory for Related Words

Directions: First review the symbols at the top of the page. The client touches the symbols in order after each group of words is read.

Objective: The client will repeat two related words after hearing a presentation of the sequence.

Kitchen Items

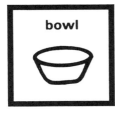
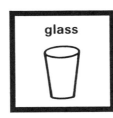
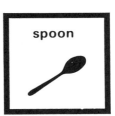
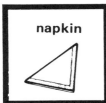

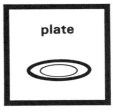

bowl - plate; _____ - _____

spoon - napkin; _____ - _____

knife - glass; _____ - _____

plate - spoon; _____ - _____

napkin - glass; _____ - _____

bowl - knife; _____ - _____

Memory for Related Words

Directions: First review the symbols at the top of the page. The client touches the symbols in order after each group of words is read.

Objective: The client will repeat two related words after hearing a presentation of the sequence.

Drinks

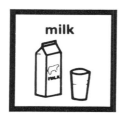  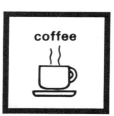

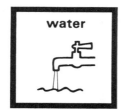 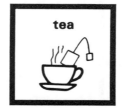 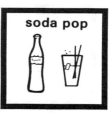

coffee - juice; _____ - _____

milk - soda; _____ - _____

tea - water; _____ - _____

coffee - milk; _____ - _____

soda - tea; _____ - _____

juice - water; _____ - _____

Memory for Related Words

Directions: First review the symbols at the top of the page. The client touches the symbols in order after each group of words is read.

Objective: The client will repeat two related words after hearing a presentation of the sequence.

Food

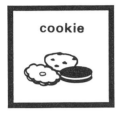

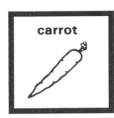

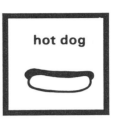

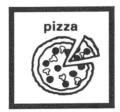

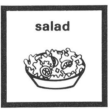

pizza - cake; _____ - _____

salad - cookie; _____ - _____

carrot - hot dog; _____ - _____

cake - salad; _____ - _____

hot dog - pizza; _____ - _____

cookie - carrot; _____ - _____

Memory for Related Words

Directions: First review the symbols at the top of the page. The client touches the symbols in order after each group of words is read.

Objective: The client will repeat two related words after hearing a presentation of the sequence.

Bathroom Items

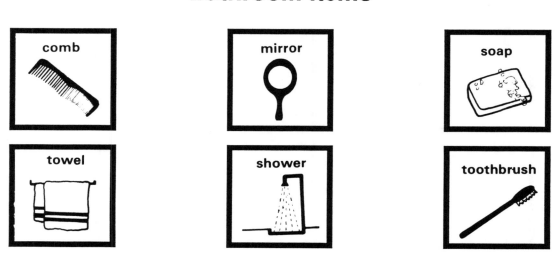

soap - toothbrush; _____ - _____

shower - comb; _____ - _____

towel - mirror; _____ - _____

toothbrush - comb; _____ - _____

towel - soap; _____ - _____

mirror - shower; _____ - _____

Memory for Related Words

Directions: First review the symbols at the top of the page. The client touches the symbols in order after each group of words is read.

Objective: The client will repeat two related words after hearing a presentation of the sequence.

Toys

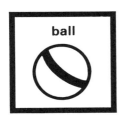

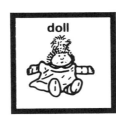

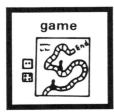

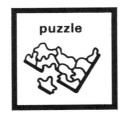

ball - puzzle; _____ - _____

crayon - game; _____ - _____

TV - doll; _____ - _____

doll - puzzle; _____ - _____

crayon - TV; _____ - _____

doll - ball; _____ - _____

Memory for Related Words

Directions: First review the symbols at the top of the page. The client touches the symbols in order after each group of words is read.

Objective: The client will repeat two related words after hearing a presentation of the sequence.

Transportation

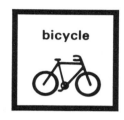

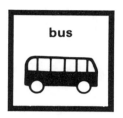

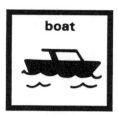

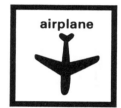

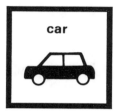

plane - bus; _____ - _____

car - boat; _____ - _____

bike - truck; _____ - _____

bus - car; _____ - _____

truck - plane; _____ - _____

boat - bike; _____ - _____

Memory for Related Words

Directions: First review the symbols at the top of the page. The client touches the symbols in order after each group of words is read.

Objective: The client will repeat three related words after hearing a presentation of the sequence.

Animals

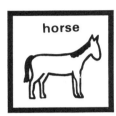
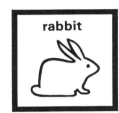
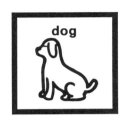
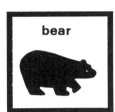
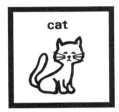
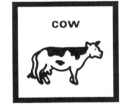
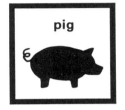
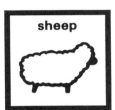

rabbit - pig - bear; _____ - _____ - _____

cow - horse - sheep; _____ - _____ - _____

dog - cat - rabbit; _____ - _____ - _____

pig - cow - horse; _____ - _____ - _____

sheep - bear - cat; _____ - _____ - _____

horse - dog - pig; _____ - _____ - _____

Memory for Related Words

Directions: First review the symbols at the top of the page. The client touches the symbols in order after each group of words is read.

Objective: The client will repeat three related words after hearing a presentation of the sequence.

School Items

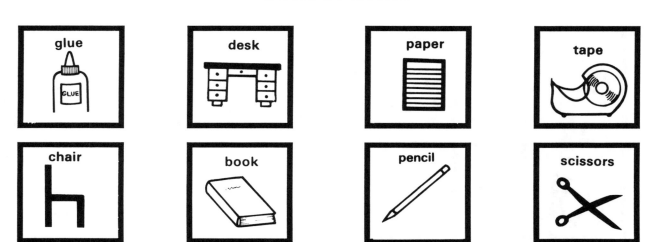

paper - books - tape; _____ - _____ - _____

scissors - desk - books; _____ - _____ - _____

pencil - tape - paper; _____ - _____ - _____

glue - chair - scissors; _____ - _____ - _____

desk - pencil - glue; _____ - _____ - _____

tape - paper - chair; _____ - _____ - _____

Memory for Related Words

Directions: First review the symbols at the top of the page. The client touches the symbols in order after each group of words is read.

Objective: The client will repeat three related words after hearing a presentation of the sequence.

Fruit

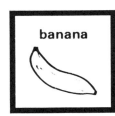

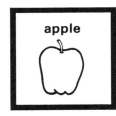

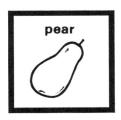

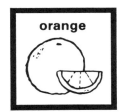

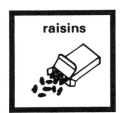

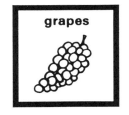

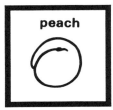

apple - pear - orange; _____ - _____ - _____

banana - grapes - peach; _____ - _____ - _____

cherry - raisins - pear; _____ - _____ - _____

orange - apple - grapes; _____ - _____ - _____

orange - peach - cherry; _____ - _____ - _____

raisins - pear - banana; _____ - _____ - _____

Memory for Related Words

Directions: First review the symbols at the top of the page. The client touches the symbols in order after each group of words is read.

Objective: The client will repeat three related words after hearing a presentation of the sequence.

Clothes

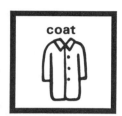
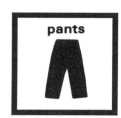
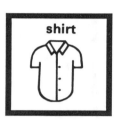
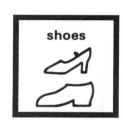

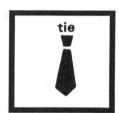

shirt - shoes - coat; _____ - _____ - _____

hat - socks - pants; _____ - _____ - _____

tie - dress - hat; _____ - _____ - _____

coat - pants - shirt; _____ - _____ - _____

shoes - dress - tie; _____ - _____ - _____

shirt - pants - socks; _____ - _____ - _____

Recalling Items to Complete a Task

Directions: First review the symbols at the top of the page. Next read through the complete list of related items in each paragraph. The client chooses a symbol to name the missing item when the partial list is repeated. Four symbols will be left over and not used as answers.

Objective: After hearing a presentation of related items needed to complete a given task, the client will recall the item omitted when all but one of the presented items are repeated.

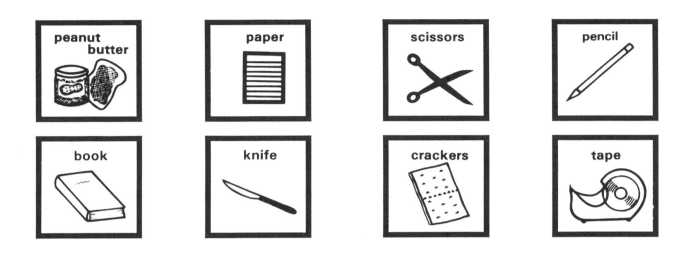

When we draw a picture, we need paper, pencil, and crayons. We need pencils and crayons. What else did I say?

When we wrap a present, we need tape, scissors, and wrapping paper. We need tape and wrapping paper. What else did I say?

When we go to school, we bring pencil, lunch, and books. We bring pencil and lunch. What else did I say?

When we make peanut butter crackers, we need peanut butter, crackers, and a knife. We need peanut butter and a knife. What else did I say?

Recalling Items to Complete a Task

Directions: First review the symbols at the top of the page. Next read through the complete list of related items in each paragraph. The client chooses a symbol to name the missing item when the partial list is repeated. Four symbols will be left over and not used as answers.

Objective: After hearing a presentation of related items needed to complete a given task, the client will recall the item omitted when all but one of the presented items are repeated.

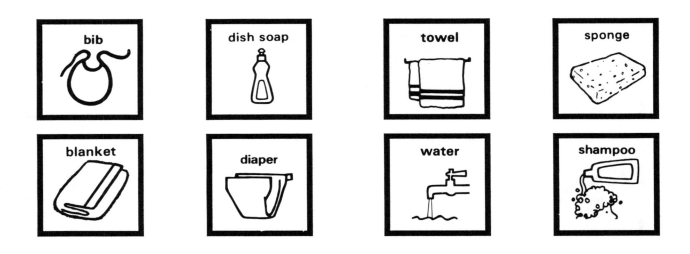

When we take the baby outside, we need extra bibs, diapers, and a bottle. We need diapers and a bottle. What else did I say?

When we go to the beach, we need towels, sandals, and a blanket. We need sandals and a blanket. What else did I say?

When I wash my hair, I need shampoo, water, and a hair dryer. I need water and a hair dryer. What else did I say?

When we do the dishes, we need a towel, dish soap, and a sponge. We need a towel and dish soap. What else did I say?

Recalling Items to Complete a Task

Directions: First review the symbols at the top of the page. Next read through the complete list of related items in each paragraph. The client chooses a symbol to name the missing item when the partial list is repeated. Four symbols will be left over and not used as answers.

Objective: After hearing a presentation of related items needed to complete a given task, the client will recall the item omitted when all but one of the presented items are repeated.

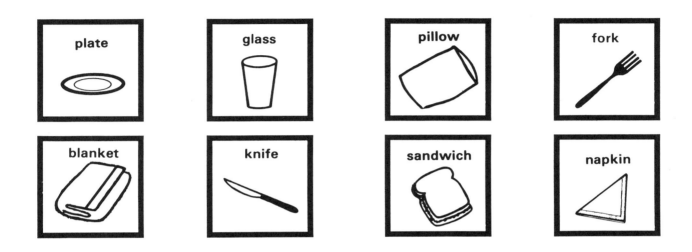

When we set the table, we need a plate, a fork, a glass, and a napkin. We need a plate, a fork, and a glass. What else did I say?

When we go on a picnic, we bring a blanket, plates, sandwiches, and napkins. We bring plates, sandwiches, and napkins. What else did I say?

When we make the bed, we need sheets, a blanket, a pillow, and a bed-spread. We need sheets, a blanket, and a bedspread. What else did I say?

When we clean up after lunch, we wash plates, glasses, forks, and knives. We wash glasses, forks, and knives. What else did I say?

Recalling Items to Complete a Task

Directions: First review the symbols at the top of the page. Next read through the complete list of related items in each paragraph. The client chooses a symbol to name the missing item when the partial list is repeated. Four symbols will be left over and not used as answers.

Objective: After hearing a presentation of related items needed to complete a given task, the client will recall the item omitted when all but one of the presented items are repeated.

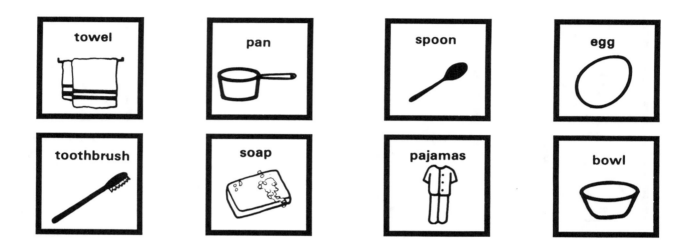

When we go camping, we bring pajamas, a toothbrush, a pan, and eggs. We need pajamas, a toothbrush, and eggs. What else did I say?

When we bake a cake, we need eggs, flour, a bowl, and a spoon. We need eggs, flour, and a spoon. What else did I say?

When we get ready for bed, we need pajamas, a toothbrush, soap, and a towel. We need a toothbrush, soap, and a towel. What else did I say?

When we take a bath, we need soap, water, a towel, and a washcloth. We need water, a towel, and a washcloth. What else did I say?

Recalling Items to Complete a Task

Directions: First review the symbols at the top of the page. Next read through the complete list of related items in each paragraph. The client chooses a symbol to name the missing item when the partial list is repeated. Four symbols will be left over and not used as answers.

Objective: After hearing a presentation of related items needed to complete a given task, the client will recall the item omitted when all but one of the presented items are repeated.

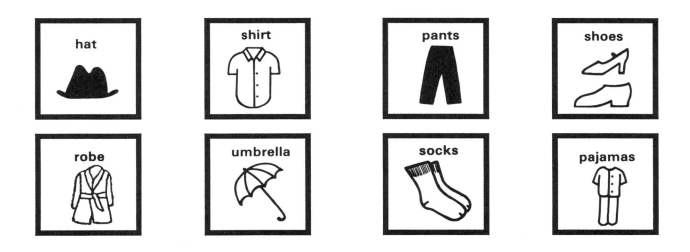

When we go outside in the rain, we need a raincoat, boots, a hat, and an umbrella. We need a raincoat, boots, and a hat. What else did I say?

When we get dressed, we wear pants, a shirt, shoes, and socks. We wear pants, a shirt, and socks. What else did I say?

When we go on a trip, we pack pajamas, a toothbrush, a shirt, and pants. We pack pajamas, a toothbrush, and a shirt. What else did I say?

When we get undressed, we wear pajamas, a bathrobe, and slippers. We wear a bathrobe and slippers. What else did I say?

Recalling Items to Complete a Task

Directions: First review the symbols at the top of the page. Next read through the complete list of related items in each paragraph. The client chooses a symbol to name the missing item when the partial list is repeated. Four symbols will be left over and not used as answers.

Objective: After hearing a presentation of related items needed to complete a given task, the client will recall the item omitted when all but one of the presented items are repeated.

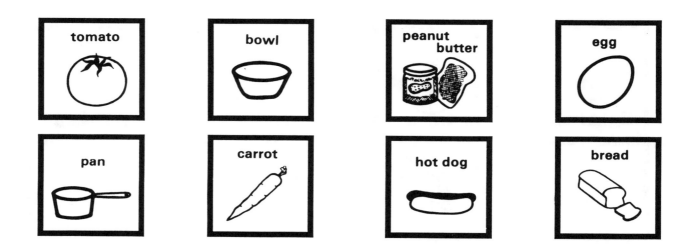

When we make a sandwich, we need bread, peanut butter, jelly, and a knife. We need peanut butter, jelly, and a knife. What else did I say?

When we make a salad, we need lettuce, tomato, carrots, and a bowl. We need lettuce, tomato, and carrots. What else did I say?

When we cook eggs, we need milk, a pan, eggs, and butter. We need milk, a pan, and butter. What else did I say?

When we have a barbecue, we eat hamburgers, hot dogs, bread, and salad. We eat hamburgers, bread, and salad. What else did I say?

Recalling One Detail from a Sentence

Directions: First review the symbols at the top of the page. The client chooses a symbol to answer a question about a sentence.

Objective: After hearing a presentation of a single sentence, the client will recall one detail in response to a "what" question.

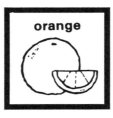

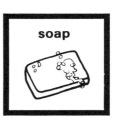

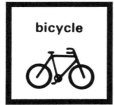

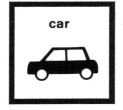

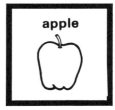

Jane likes oranges.
What does Jane like?

Barbara rides a bike.
What does Barbara ride?

Steve picks up the soap.
What does Steve pick up?

Peter buys apples.
What does Peter buy?

Dad has a new car.
What does Dad have?

Sue drops a brush.
What does Sue drop?

Recalling One Detail from a Sentence

Directions: First review the symbols at the top of the page. The client chooses a symbol to answer a question about a sentence.

Objective: After hearing a presentation of a single sentence, the client will recall one detail in response to a "what" question.

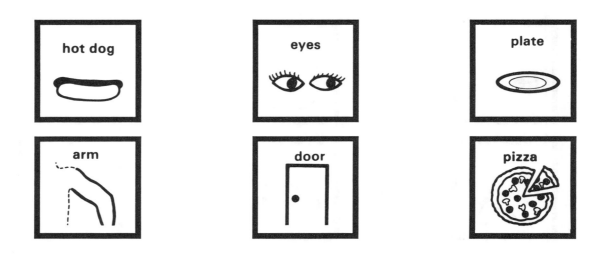

Rob hurts his arm.
What does Rob hurt?

Paul eats pizza.
What does Paul eat?

Bill closes his eyes.
What does Bill close?

Sally opens the door.
What does Sally open?

Beth cooks a hot dog.
What does Beth cook?

Mary breaks a plate.
What does Mary break?

Recalling One Detail from a Sentence

Directions: First review the symbols at the top of the page. The client chooses a symbol to answer a question about a sentence.

Objective: After hearing a presentation of a single sentence, the client will recall one detail in response to a "what" question.

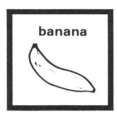

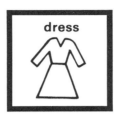

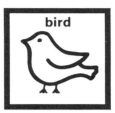

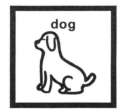

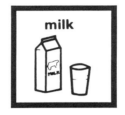

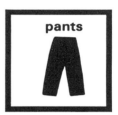

Alice rips her dress.
What does Alice rip?

Mark has a dog.
What does Mark have?

I'm wearing pants.
What am I wearing?

Jenny sees a bird.
What does Jenny see?

John peels a banana.
What does John peel?

Terry pours milk.
What does Terry pour?

Recalling One Detail from a Sentence

Directions: First review the symbols at the top of the page. The client chooses a symbol to answer a question about a sentence.

Objective: After hearing a presentation of a single sentence, the client will recall one detail in response to a "what" question.

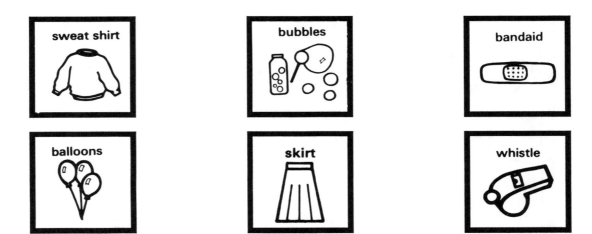

Bobby blew a whistle.
What did Bobby blow?

Debbie popped a balloon.
What did Debbie pop?

Nicholas bought a bottle of bubbles.
What did Nicholas buy?

I put a bandaid on my cut.
What did I put on?

Claire wore a red skirt.
What did Claire wear?

Doug has a new sweatshirt.
What does Doug have?

Recalling One Detail from a Sentence

Directions: First review the symbols at the top of the page. The client chooses a symbol to answer a question about a sentence.

Objective: After hearing a presentation of a single sentence, the client will recall one detail in response to a "where" question.

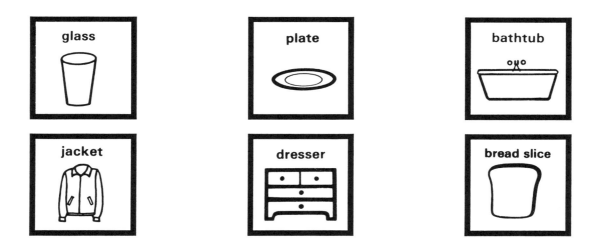

The cheese is on the bread.
Where is the cheese?

The hamburger is on the plate.
Where is the hamburger?

The soap fell in the bathtub.
Where did the soap fall?

The money is in my jacket.
Where is the money?

The socks are in my dresser.
Where are the socks?

The juice is in the glass.
Where is the juice?

Recalling One Detail from a Sentence

Directions: First review the symbols at the top of the page. The client chooses a symbol to answer a question about a sentence.

Objective: After hearing a presentation of a single sentence, the client will recall one detail in response to a "where" question.

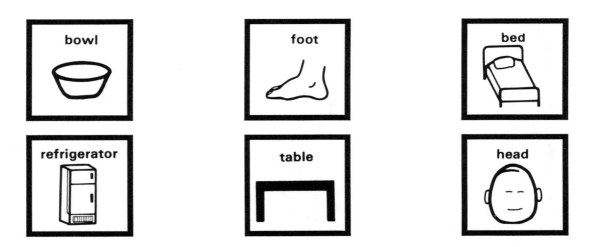

The pudding is in the refrigerator.
Where is the pudding?

A hat is on my head.
Where is my hat?

The spoon is in the bowl.
Where is the spoon?

A lamp is on the table.
Where is the lamp?

My shoes are under my bed.
Where are my shoes?

My socks are on my feet.
Where are my socks?

Recalling One Detail from a Sentence

Directions: First review the symbols at the top of the page. The client chooses a symbol to answer a question about a sentence.

Objective: After hearing a presentation of a single sentence, the client will recall one detail in response to a "where" question.

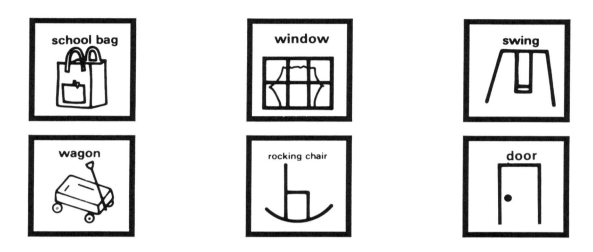

The curtains are on the window.
Where are the curtains?

I put my books in my school bag.
Where did I put my books?

Davie sat on the wagon.
Where did Davie sit?

Stacy fell asleep in the rocking chair.
Where did Stacy fall asleep?

Bill is playing on the swing.
Where is Bill playing?

I hung a wreath on the door.
Where did I hang a wreath?

Recalling One Detail from a Sentence

Directions: First review the symbols at the top of the page. The client chooses a symbol to answer a question about a sentence.

Objective: After hearing a presentation of a single sentence, the client will recall one detail in response to a "where" question.

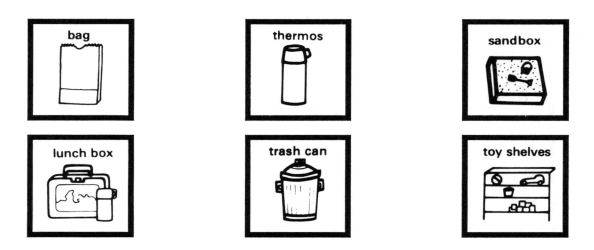

I packed my sandwich in my lunchbox.
Where did I pack my sandwich?

I threw the candy wrapper in the trash can.
Where did I throw the candy wrapper?

I left the shovel in the sandbox.
Where did I leave the shovel?

I poured the milk in my thermos.
Where did I pour the milk?

I put my car on the toy shelf.
Where did I put my car?

The cashier put my groceries in a bag.
Where did the cashier put my groceries?

Recalling Details from a Sentence

Directions: First review the symbols at the top of the page. The client chooses two symbols to answer a question about a sentence.

Objective: After hearing a presentation of a single sentence, the client will recall two details in response to a "what" question.

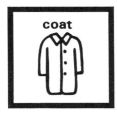
coat

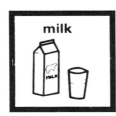
milk

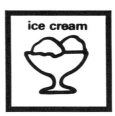
ice cream

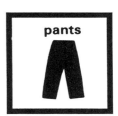
pants

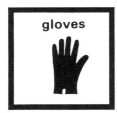
gloves

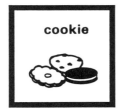
cookie

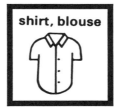
shirt, blouse

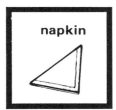
napkin

Tom eats ice cream and cookies.
What does Tom eat?

Ray wears a shirt and pants.
What does Ray wear?

Sheryl puts on her coat and gloves.
What does Sheryl put on?

Kathy buys new pants and a coat.
What does Kathy buy?

Put the cookies and milk on the table.
What goes on the table?

Take out the ice cream and napkins.
What do I take out?

Recalling Details from a Sentence

Directions: First review the symbols at the top of the page. The client chooses two symbols to answer a question about a sentence.

Objective: After hearing a presentation of a single sentence, the client will recall two details in response to a "what" question.

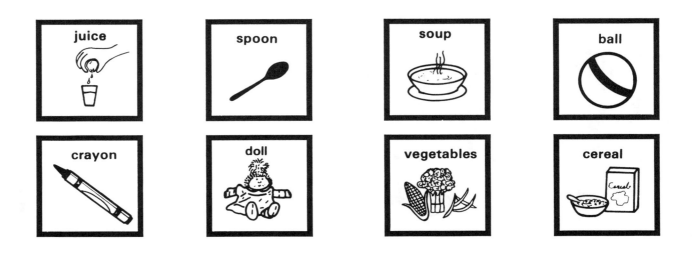

The soup and vegetables are too hot.
What are too hot?

Here's the cereal and juice for breakfast.
What's for breakfast?

Let's play with the doll and ball.
What are we playing with?

The crayons and doll are in the closet.
What are in the closet?

Take the cereal and spoon.
What do I take?

Put away the soup and juice.
What do I put away?

Recalling Details from a Sentence

Directions: First review the symbols at the top of the page. The client chooses two symbols to answer a question about a sentence.

Objective: After hearing a presentation of a single sentence, the client will recall two details in response to a "what" question.

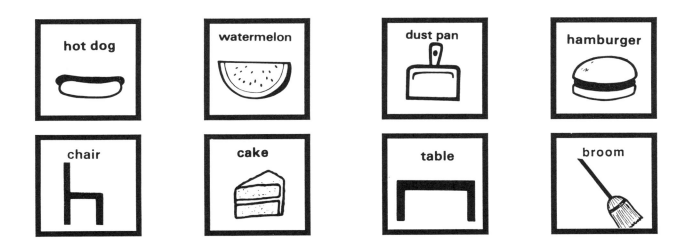

Put the hot dogs and hamburgers on the grill.
What do I put on the grill?

We had watermelon and cake for dessert.
What did we have for dessert?

Sandy put away the dust pan and broom.
What did Sandy put away?

Maria dusted the chair and table.
What did Maria dust?

I put the hot dogs and watermelon on the counter.
What did I put on the counter?

The chair and broom are near the table.
What are near the table?

Recalling Details from a Sentence

Directions: First review the symbols at the top of the page. The client chooses two symbols to answer a question about a sentence.

Objective: After hearing a presentation of a single sentence, the client will recall two details in response to a "what" question.

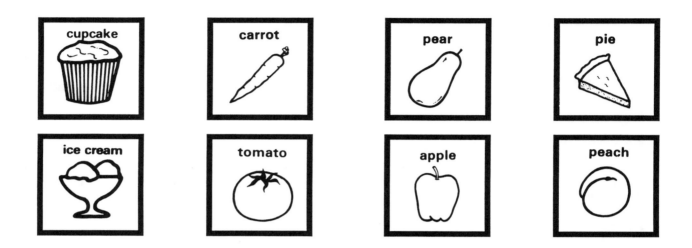

Sonya baked cupcakes and a pie.
What did Sonya bake?

We planted carrots and tomato plants.
What did we plant?

Paul served cupcakes and ice cream at his party.
What did Paul serve?

We put peaches and pears in the pie.
What did we put in the pie?

Jane picked tomatoes and peaches at the farm.
What did Jane pick?

Take the carrots and apples out of the refrigerator.
What do I take out of the refrigerator?

Recalling Details from a Short Story

Directions: First review the symbols at the top of the page. Then read the short story. The client chooses symbols to answer questions related to the story. Encourage the client to answer with two word phrases when appropriate. Some symbols may be left over and not used as answers.

Objective: After hearing a presentation of a short story, the client will recall facts from the story by answering questions.

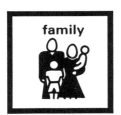

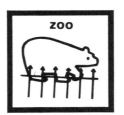

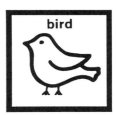

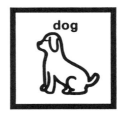

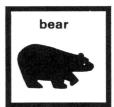

The Smith family goes to the zoo. They see bears and cages full of birds.

Where do the Smiths go?

What do they see at the zoo?

Directions: Reread the story. To retell the story, the client chooses symbols to fill in the blanks as the phrases below are read. Some clients may need questions such as "What happened next?" or "Who did that?" to prompt their answers.

Objective: The client will retell the story by filling in the blanks.

The Smith _____ goes to the _____. They see

_____ and cages full of _____.

Recalling Details from a Short Story

Directions: First review the symbols at the top of the page. Then read the short story. The client chooses symbols to answer questions related to the story. Encourage the client to answer with two word phrases when appropriate. Some symbols may be left over and not used as answers.

Objective: After hearing a presentation of a short story, the client will recall facts from the story by answering questions.

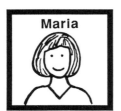 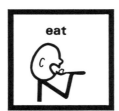 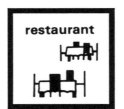 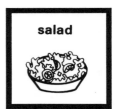

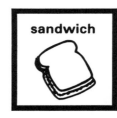 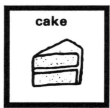

Maria goes to the restaurant. She eats a sandwich and cake.

Where does Maria go?

What does she do at the restaurant?

What does she eat?

Who goes to the restaurant?

Directions: Reread the story. To retell the story, the client chooses symbols to fill in the blanks as the phrases below are read. Some clients may need questions such as "What happened next?" or "Who did that?" to prompt their answers.

Objective: The client will retell the story by filling in the blanks.

Maria goes to the _____. She _____ a _____

and _____.

Recalling Details from a Short Story

Directions: First review the symbols at the top of the page. Then read the short story. The client chooses symbols to answer questions related to the story. Encourage the client to answer with two word phrases when appropriate. Some symbols may be left over and not used as answers.

Objective: After hearing a presentation of a short story, the client will recall facts from the story by answering questions.

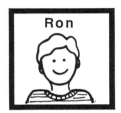 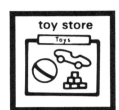 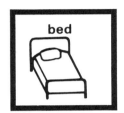 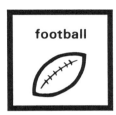

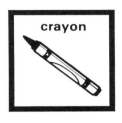 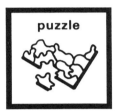

Ron went to the toy store. He bought a box of crayons and a

puzzle.

Where did Ron go?

What did he buy?

Who went to the store?

Directions: Reread the story. To retell the story, the client chooses symbols to fill in the blanks as the phrases below are read. Some clients may need questions such as "What happened next?" or "Who did that?" to prompt their answers.

Objective: The client will retell the story by filling in the blanks.

Ron went to the _____. He bought a box of _____

and a _____.

Recalling Details from a Short Story

Directions: First review the symbols at the top of the page. Then read the short story. The client chooses symbols to answer questions related to the story. Encourage the client to answer with two word phrases when appropriate. Some symbols may be left over and not used as answers.

Objective: After hearing a presentation of a short story, the client will recall facts from the story by answering questions.

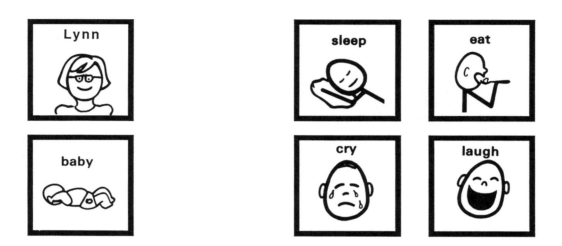

Lynn has a new baby brother. He sleeps and cries a lot. Lynn likes to make him laugh.

Who is new in Lynn's family?

What does he do most of the time?

What does Lynn make the baby do?

Directions: Reread the story. To retell the story, the client chooses symbols to fill in the blanks as the phrases below are read. Some clients may need questions such as "What happened next?" or "Who did that?" to prompt their answers.

Objective: The client will retell the story by filling in the blanks.

Lynn has a new _____ brother. He _____ and

_____ a lot. Lynn likes to make him _____.

Recalling Details from a Short Story

Directions: First review the symbols at the top of the page. Then read the short story. The client chooses symbols to answer questions related to the story. Encourage the client to answer with two word phrases when appropriate. Some symbols may be left over and not used as answers.

Objective: After hearing a presentation of a short story, the client will recall facts from the story by answering questions.

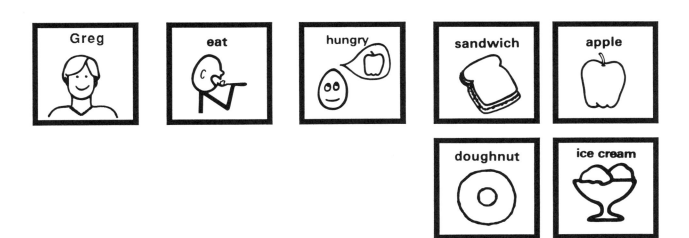

Greg feels very hungry. He eats two sandwiches, a dish of ice cream, and two doughnuts.

Who is hungry?

What does Greg do?

What does he eat?

Directions: Reread the story. To retell the story, the client chooses symbols to fill in the blanks as the phrases below are read. Some clients may need questions such as "What happened next?" or "Who did that?" to prompt their answers.

Objective: The client will retell the story by filling in the blanks.

_____ feels very _____. He eats two _____, a

dish of _____, and two _____.

Recalling Details from a Short Story

Directions: First review the symbols at the top of the page. Then read the short story. The client chooses symbols to answer questions related to the story. Encourage the client to answer with two word phrases when appropriate. Some symbols may be left over and not used as answers.

Objective: After hearing a presentation of a short story, the client will recall facts from the story by answering questions.

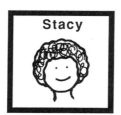

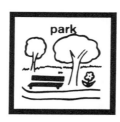

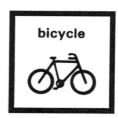

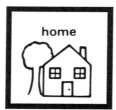

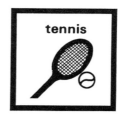

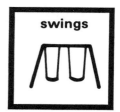

Stacy rides her bike to the park. She plays on the swings. Then she goes home.

What does Stacy ride?

Where does she go on her bike?

What does she play on at the park?

Who rides her bike?

Directions: Reread the story. To retell the story, the client chooses symbols to fill in the blanks as the phrases below are read. Some clients may need questions such as "What happened next?" or "Who did that?" to prompt their answers.

Objective: The client will retell the story by filling in the blanks.

Stacy rides her _____ to the _____. She plays on the _____. Then she goes _____.

Recalling Details from a Short Story

Directions: First review the symbols at the top of the page. Then read the short story. The client chooses symbols to answer questions related to the story. Encourage the client to answer with two word phrases when appropriate. Some symbols may be left over and not used as answers.

Objective: After hearing a presentation of a short story, the client will recall facts from the story by answering questions.

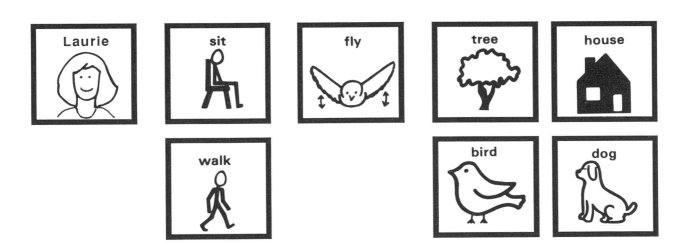

Laurie takes a walk. She sees trees, houses, and birds flying.

What does Laurie do?

What does she see?

What are the birds doing?

Who takes a walk?

Directions: Reread the story. To retell the story, the client chooses symbols to fill in the blanks as the phrases below are read. Some clients may need questions such as "What happened next?" or "Who did that?" to prompt their answers.

Objective: The client will retell the story by filling in the blanks.

Laurie takes a _____. She sees _____,

_____, and birds _____.

Recalling Details from a Short Story

Directions: First review the symbols at the top of the page. Then read the short story. The client chooses symbols to answer questions related to the story. Encourage the client to answer with two word phrases when appropriate. Some symbols may be left over and not used as answers.

Objective: After hearing a presentation of a short story, the client will recall facts from the story by answering questions.

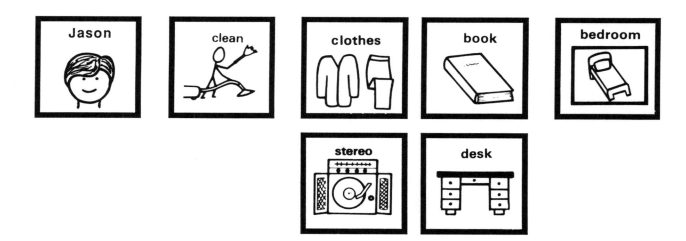

Jason has to clean up his bedroom. He hangs up his clothes and puts his books on his desk.

What does Jason have to do?

What room does he have to clean?

What does he hang up?

Where does he put his books?

Directions: Reread the story. To retell the story, the client chooses symbols to fill in the blanks as the phrases below are read. Some clients may need questions such as "What happened next?" or "Who did that?" to prompt their answers.

Objective: The client will retell the story by filling in the blanks.

Jason has to _____ up his room. He hangs up his

_____ and puts his _____ on his _____.

Recalling Details from a Short Story

Directions: First review the symbols at the top of the page. Then read the short story. The client chooses symbols to answer questions related to the story. Encourage the client to answer with two word phrases when appropriate. Some symbols may be left over and not used as answers.

Objective: After hearing a presentation of a short story, the client will recall facts from the story by answering questions.

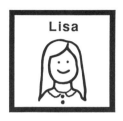 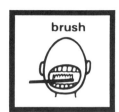 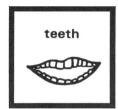 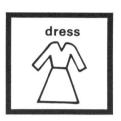 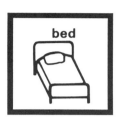

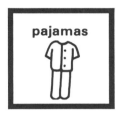 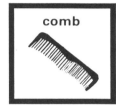 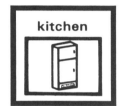

Lisa is going to bed. She must brush her teeth and put on her pajamas.

Where is Lisa going?

What does she do to her teeth?

What does she put on before going to bed?

Who goes to bed?

Directions: Reread the story. To retell the story, the client chooses symbols to fill in the blanks as the phrases below are read. Some clients may need questions such as "What happened next?" or "Who did that?" to prompt their answers.

Objective: The client will retell the story by filling in the blanks.

Lisa is going to _____. She must brush her _____ and put on her _____.

Recalling Details from a Short Story

Directions: First review the symbols at the top of the page. Then read the short story. The client chooses symbols to answer questions related to the story. Encourage the client to answer with two word phrases when appropriate. Some symbols may be left over and not used as answers.

Objective: After hearing a presentation of a short story, the client will recall facts from the story by answering questions.

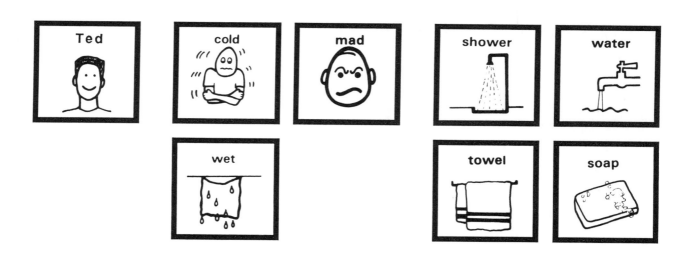

Ted is the last person in his house to take a shower. He feels mad because the water is so cold, the towels are all wet, and there's no more soap.

What does Ted do?

How does he feel?

How does the water feel?

What's all wet?

Did they run out of something? What?

Directions: Reread the story. To retell the story, the client chooses symbols to fill in the blanks as the phrases below are read. Some clients may need questions such as "What happened next?" or "Who did that?" to prompt their answers.

Objective: The client will retell the story by filling in the blanks.

Ted is the last person in his house to take a _____. He

feels _____ because the water is _____, the towels

are all _____, and there's no more _____.

Recalling Details from a Short Story

Directions: First review the symbols at the top of the page. Then read the short story. The client chooses symbols to answer questions related to the story. Encourage the client to answer with two word phrases when appropriate. Some symbols may be left over and not used as answers.

Objective: After hearing a presentation of a short story, the client will recall facts from the story by answering questions.

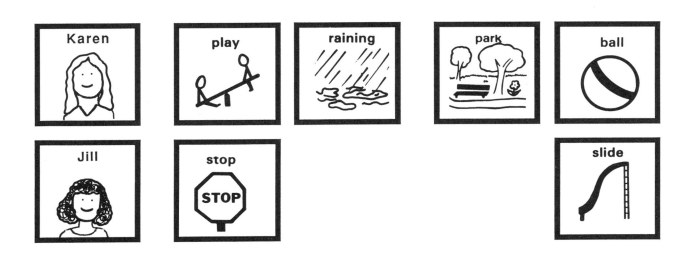

Karen and Jill are playing at the park. It starts to rain. Karen and Jill wait under the slide and stay dry until it stops raining.

What are Karen and Jill doing?

Where are they playing?

What happens when they are playing?

Where do they go to stay dry?

When will they come out from under the slide?

Directions: Reread the story. To retell the story, the client chooses symbols to fill in the blanks as the phrases below are read. Some clients may need questions such as "What happened next?" or "Who did that?" to prompt their answers.

Objective: The client will retell the story by filling in the blanks.

Karen and Jill are _____ at the _____. It starts to

_____. Karen and Jill wait under the _____ and stay

dry until it stops _____.

Recalling Details from a Short Story

Directions: First review the symbols at the top of the page. Then read the short story. The client chooses symbols to answer questions related to the story. Encourage the client to answer with two word phrases when appropriate. Some symbols may be left over and not used as answers.

Objective: After hearing a presentation of a short story, the client will recall facts from the story by answering questions.

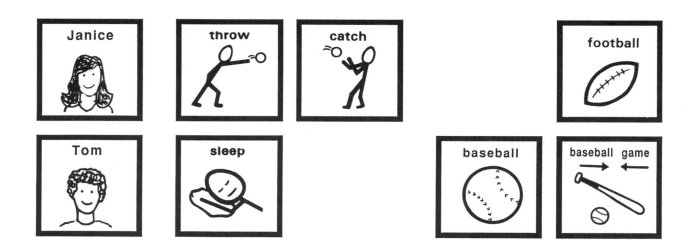

One very sunny day, Tom and Janice go to a baseball game. The batter hits a high ball. Janice looks up and catches the ball. She shows the ball to Tom, but he's asleep.

Where do Tom and Janice go?

What does Janice do during the game?

What does she catch?

What does Tom do?

Directions: Reread the story. To retell the story, the client chooses symbols to fill in the blanks as the phrases below are read. Some clients may need questions such as "What happened next?" or "Who did that?" to prompt their answers.

Objective: The client will retell the story by filling in the blanks.

One very sunny day Tom and Janice go to a _____. The batter hits a high ball. Janice looks up and _____ the _____. She shows the ball to _____, but he's _____.

Recalling Details from a Short Story

Directions: First review the symbols at the top of the page. Then read the short story. The client chooses symbols to answer questions related to the story. Encourage the client to answer with two word phrases when appropriate. Some symbols may be left over and not used as answers.

Objective: After hearing a presentation of a short story, the client will recall facts from the story by answering questions.

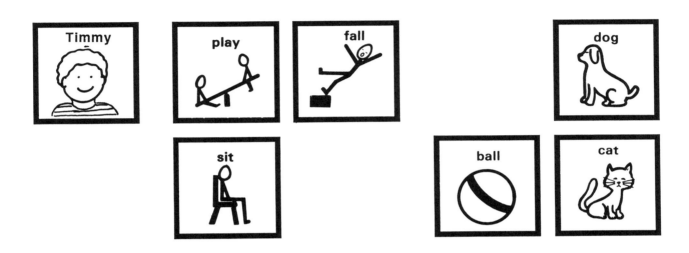

Timmy and his dog are playing with a ball. Timmy tries to catch the ball but he falls over a rock. The dog gets the ball.

What are they playing with?

Who gets the ball?

Why doesn't Timmy get the ball?

Who falls?

Directions: Reread the story. To retell the story, the client chooses symbols to fill in the blanks as the phrases below are read. Some clients may need questions such as "What happened next?" or "Who did that?" to prompt their answers.

Objective: The client will retell the story by filling in the blanks.

Timmy and his _____ are _____. Timmy tries to

catch the _____ but he _____ over a rock. The

_____ gets the _____.

Recalling Details from a Short Story

Directions: First review the symbols at the top of the page. Then read the short story. The client chooses symbols to answer questions related to the story. Encourage the client to answer with two word phrases when appropriate. Some symbols may be left over and not used as answers.

Objective: After hearing a presentation of a short story, the client will recall facts from the story by answering questions.

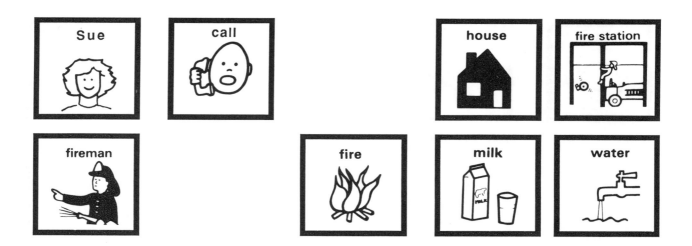

Sue is surprised to see the corner house is on fire. She calls the fire station. In a minute she hears the fire engine coming. Three firemen rush out and spray water to put out the fire.

What does Sue see?

What is on fire?

Who does Sue call?

Who comes in the fire engine?

What do the firemen spray?

Directions: Reread the story. To retell the story, the client chooses symbols to fill in the blanks as the phrases below are read. Some clients may need questions such as "What happened next?" or "Who did that?" to prompt their answers.

Objective: The client will retell the story by filling in the blanks.

Sue is surprised to see that the corner _____ is on _____. She calls the _____. In a minute she hears the fire engine coming. Three _____ rush out and spray _____ to put out the _____.

Recalling Details from a Short Story

Directions: First review the symbols at the top of the page. Then read the short story. The client chooses symbols to answer questions related to the story. Encourage the client to answer with two word phrases when appropriate. Some symbols may be left over and not used as answers.

Objective: After hearing a presentation of a short story, the client will recall facts from the story by answering questions.

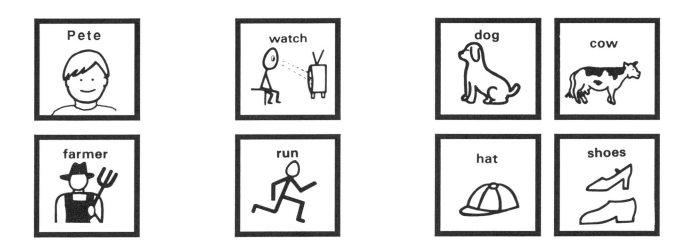

Pete goes to visit the farmer next door. He stands in the fields and watches the cows. The farmer's dog takes Pete's hat and runs away.

Who goes to the farm?

Who does Pete go to visit?

What animal does Pete watch at the farm?

What is Pete missing?

Who took Pete's hat?

What does the dog do next?

Directions: Reread the story. To retell the story, the client chooses symbols to fill in the blanks as the phrases below are read. Some clients may need questions such as "What happened next?" or "Who did that?" to prompt their answers.

Objective: The client will retell the story by filling in the blanks.

Pete goes to visit the _____ next door. He stands in the fields and _____ the _____. The farmer's _____ takes Pete's _____ and _____ away.

Recalling Details from a Short Story

Directions: First review the symbols at the top of the page. Then read the short story. The client chooses symbols to answer questions related to the story. Encourage the client to answer with two word phrases when appropriate. Some symbols may be left over and not used as answers.

Objective: After hearing a presentation of a short story, the client will recall facts from the story by answering questions.

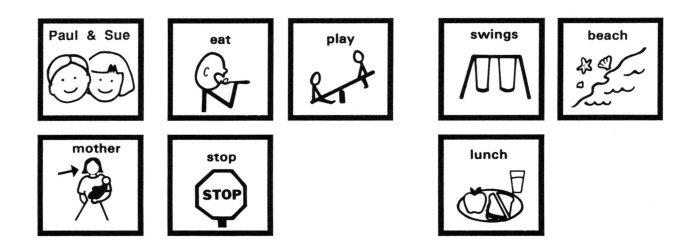

Paul and Sue are playing in the sand at the beach. "It's time for lunch," yells Mom. They stop playing.

What are Paul and Sue doing?

Where are they?

Why do they stop playing?

Who calls them?

Directions: Reread the story. To retell the story, the client chooses symbols to fill in the blanks as the phrases below are read. Some clients may need questions such as "What happened next?" or "Who did that?" to prompt their answers.

Objective: The client will retell the story by filling in the blanks.

Paul and Sue are _____ in the sand at the _____.

"It's time for _____," yells _____. They stop

_____.

Recalling Details from a Short Story

Directions: First review the symbols at the top of the page. Then read the short story. The client chooses symbols to answer questions related to the story. Encourage the client to answer with two word phrases when appropriate. Some symbols may be left over and not used as answers.

Objective: After hearing a presentation of a short story, the client will recall facts from the story by answering questions.

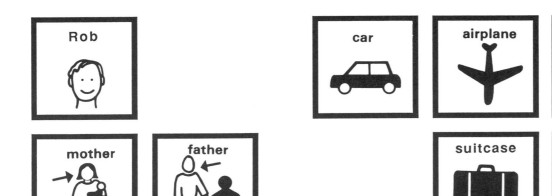

Rob drives his car to the airport. He waits for his father to get off the airplane. His father is carrying a suitcase and presents as he walks toward Rob.

Who drives to the airport?

What does Rob drive to the airport?

Who does Rob wait for at the airport?

How does his father get to the airport?

What is Rob's father carrying?

Directions: Reread the story. To retell the story, the client chooses symbols to fill in the blanks as the phrases below are read. Some clients may need questions such as "What happened next?" or "Who did that?" to prompt their answers.

Objective: The client will retell the story by filling in the blanks.

Rob drives his _____ to the airport. He waits for his

_____ to get off the _____. His father is carrying a

_____ and _____.

Recalling Details from a Short Story

Directions: First review the symbols at the top of the page. Then read the short story. The client chooses symbols to answer questions related to the story. Encourage the client to answer with two word phrases when appropriate. Some symbols may be left over and not used as answers.

Objective: After hearing a presentation of a short story, the client will recall facts from the story by answering questions.

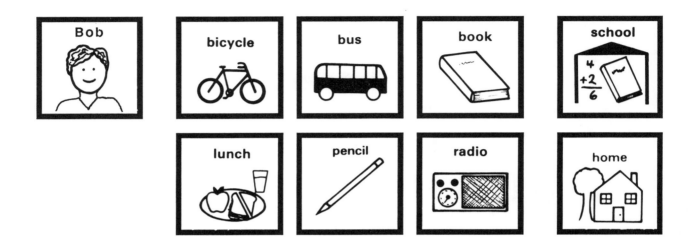

Bob waits for the bus to take him to school. He remembers his lunch, a pencil, and his books.

Who goes to school?

Where is Bob going?

How does he get to school?

What does Bob take to school?

Directions: Reread the story. To retell the story, the client chooses symbols to fill in the blanks as the phrases below are read. Some clients may need questions such as "What happened next?" or "Who did that?" to prompt their answers.

Objective: The client will retell the story by filling in the blanks.

Bob waits for the _____ to take him to _____. He

remembers to bring his _____, a _____, and his

_____.

Recalling Details from a Short Story

Directions: First review the symbols at the top of the page. Then read the short story. The client chooses symbols to answer questions related to the story. Encourage the client to answer with two word phrases when appropriate. Some symbols may be left over and not used as answers.

Objective: After hearing a presentation of a short story, the client will recall facts from the story by answering questions.

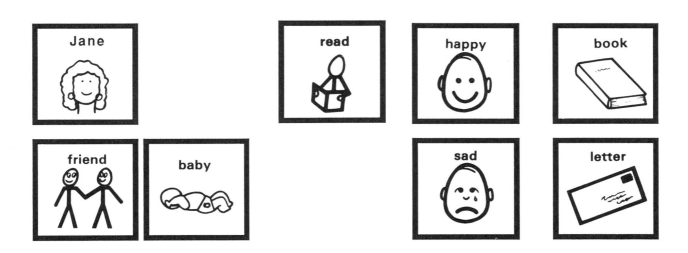

Jane takes a letter out of the mailbox and reads it. The letter is from her old friend Bill. Jane is very happy.

What does Jane get?

What does she do with the letter?

Who is the letter from?

How does Jane feel?

Directions: Reread the story. To retell the story, the client chooses symbols to fill in the blanks as the phrases below are read. Some clients may need questions such as "What happened next?" or "Who did that?" to prompt their answers.

Objective: The client will retell the story by filling in the blanks.

Jane takes a _____ out of the mailbox and _____ it.

The letter is from her old _____ Bill. Jane is very

_____.

Recalling Details from a Short Story

Directions: First review the symbols at the top of the page. Then read the short story. The client chooses symbols to answer questions related to the story. Encourage the client to answer with two word phrases when appropriate. Some symbols may be left over and not used as answers.

Objective: After hearing a presentation of a short story, the client will recall facts from the story by answering questions.

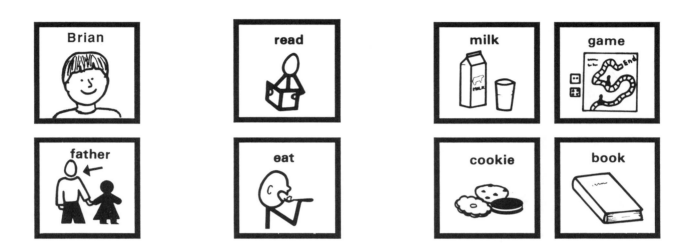

"Brian, please bring some milk and cookies," said Dad. "Then

we'll finish our snack and I'll read you a story"

Who is talking to Brian?

What does Dad ask Brian to bring?

What will they do with the snack?

What will they do after they eat the snack?

Directions: Reread the story. To retell the story, the client chooses symbols to fill in the blanks as the phrases below are read. Some clients may need questions such as "What happened next?" or "Who did that?" to prompt their answers.

Objective: The client will retell the story by filling in the blanks.

"Brian, please bring some _____ and _____," said

Dad. "Then we'll finish our snack and I'll _____ you a

_____."

284

Following Complex Directions

Directions: First review the symbols at the top of the page. The client touches the symbols in order after each sentence is read. Some competency in categorization is recommended.

Objective: The client will recall (touch) the items in the order designated by the sentence.

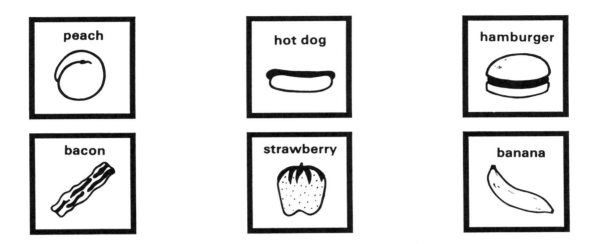

Touch only one fruit and one meat.

Before you touch hot dog, touch peach.

Touch banana after you touch bacon.

Touch a meat after you touch strawberry and peach.

Touch a fruit after you touch hamburger.

Touch hot dog and peach before you touch bacon.

Following Complex Directions

Directions: First review the symbols at the top of the page. The client touches the symbols in order after each sentence is read. Some competency in categorization is recommended.

Objective: The client will recall (touch) the items in the order designated by the sentence.

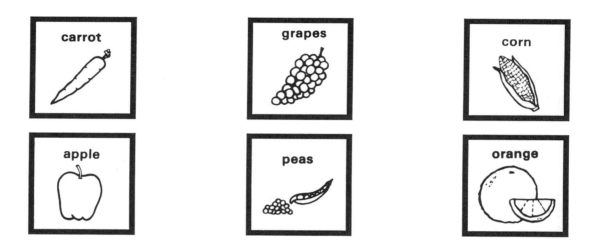

Touch all of the vegetables.

Touch carrot after you touch apple.

Touch a fruit before you touch corn.

Touch orange and peas after you touch grapes.

After you touch apple, touch corn.

Touch only one fruit and vegetable.

Following Complex Directions

Directions: First review the symbols at the top of the page. The client touches the symbols in order after each sentence is read. Some competency in categorization is recommended.

Objective: The client will recall (touch) the items in the order designated by the sentence.

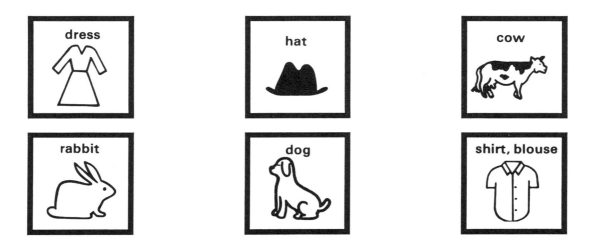

Touch all the animals.

Touch hat after you touch dog and dress.

Touch rabbit before you touch shirt.

Touch cow after you touch dog.

Touch an animal before you touch shirt.

Touch dress and cow before you touch hat.

Following Complex Directions

Directions: First review the symbols at the top of the page. The client touches the symbols in order after each sentence is read. Some competency in categorization is recommended.

Objective: The client will recall (touch) the items in the order designated by the sentence.

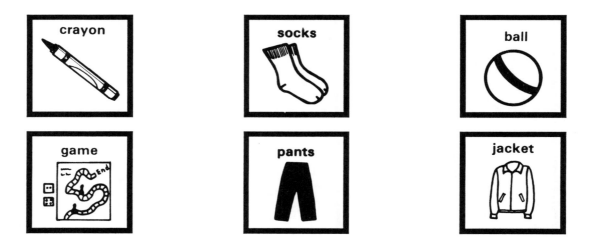

Touch all the clothes.

After you touch socks, touch game.

Touch ball and jacket before you touch pants.

Touch a toy after you touch jacket.

Touch game and crayon after you touch socks.

Touch ball before you touch crayon.

Following Complex Directions

Directions: First review the symbols at the top of the page. The client touches the symbols in order after each sentence is read. Some competency in categorization is recommended.

Objective: The client will recall (touch) the items in the order designated by the sentence.

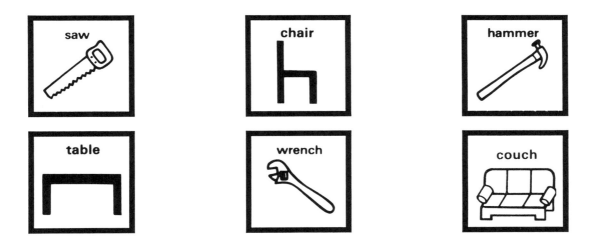

Touch all the tools.

Touch a piece of furniture before you touch saw.

Touch hammer after you touch something to sit on.

Touch table and chair before you touch wrench.

Touch couch before you touch a tool.

After you touch couch, touch saw.

Following Complex Directions

Directions: First review the symbols at the top of the page. The client touches the symbols in order after each sentence is read. Some competency in categorization is recommended.

Objective: The client will recall (touch) the items in the order designated by the sentence.

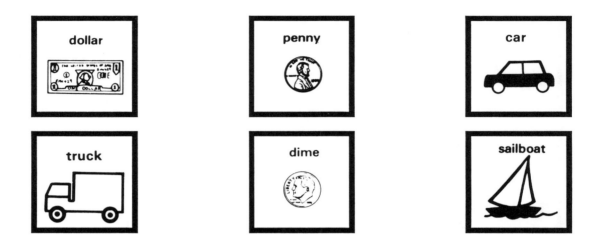

Touch all the vehicles.

Touch truck after you touch any kind of money.

Before you touch car, touch penny.

Touch only one coin and one vehicle.

Touch dollar and truck after you touch sailboat.

After you touch dime, touch car.

ABOUT THE *PICTURE COMMUNICATION SYMBOLS*

The Picture Communication Symbols (PCS) were specifically designed for the non-speech population. There are over 700 symbols in Book I, 1,100 symbols in Book II, and an additional 1400 symbols in Book III. The symbols are provided in 1" and 2" sizes and may be copied on copying machines. Since their development, the symbols have been used with various types of disabilities involving a wide range of activities. The following are a few samples of symbols besides those contained in this book:

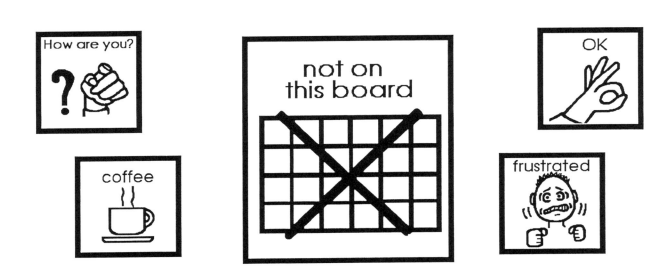

Various books and communication boards are available from the Mayer-Johnson Co. to display the PCS.

THE *PICTURE COMMUNICATION SYMBOLS* (PCS)
IN OTHER FORMATS

COMPUTER PROGRAMS
The PCS are available on computer discs for the Macintosh, Apple II series, and PC computers. Ideal for making communication boards, overlays of all sizes, or your own instructional materials. Programs also allow easy translation of the PCS to other languages.

STAMPS AND STICKERS
The PCS are also available in both a stamp and sticker format, color-coded or black and white.

THE PCS WORDLESS EDITION
Both the Book I and Book II symbols are included in this book. Each symbol comes in 3/4", 1", and 2" size. Space is provided to write a word above each symbol, or the symbols can be used by themselves without any word above. Ideal for many communication aides or for translating the symbols into other languages.

OTHER ACTIVITY/INSTRUCTIONAL MATERIALS AVAILABLE USING THE
PICTURE COMMUNICATION SYMBOLS

THIS IS THE ONE I WANT
A 172 page fun, color, cut, and paste activity book designed for the non-speech or limited speech students. Thirty-four activities with accompanying question sheets and communication boards give many opportunities for symbol communication. Activities may be easily adapted so that the instructor does the actual cutting and pasting for the physically handicapped client.

STORIES ABOUT ME!
Here's a chance for clients of all ages to "write" and "read" stories about themselves. Each story is four or five lines long and is made primarily with the Picture Communication Symbols. The client fills in the blanks to personalize each story. Over 200 reproducible stories are designed around home and family, school, activities, sports, holidays, weather and health and augmentative aids. A great way to encourage language with clients who have limited expressive language abilities.

SIMPLY SILLY ABOUT SYNTAX
Over 270 pages of silly exercises to put fun into teaching language. Three and four word sentence structures are practiced using everyday vocabulary. No reading or speaking is necessary by the client as picture symbols are used. Get to know Silly Sue, the DoRight Twins, and Maxi the Dog!

WHAT'S IN YOUR HOME?
WHAT'S IN YOUR COMMUNITY?
Low-level workbooks that each student may keep as their own. The books are designed for students who need practice with everyday vocabulary, such as "chair", "store", and "bedroom". Each workbook includes discussion sheets, study sheets, vocabulary worksheets, unit reviews, and unit review worksheets.

LIFE EXPERIENCES KIT
A unique set of eleven different "lesson plans" designed for non-speech or limited speech students. The plans and materials teach specific daily life activity skills, such as "Make Juice", "Wash Hands", and "Go Restaurant". Included are symbol instructions sheets and communication boards.

PICTURE SYMBOL LOTTO
This special lotto game is set up in color coded sections of verbs, adjectives and nouns. An excellent opportunity to reinforce common vocabulary and color-coding cues used on communication boards.

HOLIDAY KIT
The Holiday Kit is a set of low level materials based on holidays designed to stimulate enthusiasm, interest, and conversation in your clients. The kit includes a folder and 9 pre-made communication boards in both 1" and 2" sizes. Symbol masters for an additional 15 holidays are also included.

For further information on these products and others, please call or write for a free brochure.

Mayer-Johnson Co.
P.O. Box 1579
Solana Beach, CA 92075
U.S.A.

Phone (619) 550-0084
Fax (619) 550-0449